Prevention and Management of Complications from Gynecologic Surgery

Guest Editor

HOWARD T. SHARP, MD

OBSTETRICS AND GYNECOLOGY CLINICS OF NORTH AMERICA

www.obgyn.theclinics.com

Consulting Editor
WILLIAM F. RAYBURN, MD, MBA

September 2010 • Volume 37 • Number 3

SAUNDERS an imprint of ELSEVIER, Inc.

W.B. SAUNDERS COMPANY
A Division of Elsevier Inc.

Elsevier, Inc. • 1600 John F. Kennedy Blvd. • Suite 1800 • Philadelphia, PA 19103-2899

http://www.theclinics.com

OBSTETRICS AND GYNECOLOGY CLINICS OF NORTH AMERICA Volume 37, Number 3
September 2010 ISSN 0889-8545, ISBN-13: 978-1-4377-2470-7

Editor: Carla Holloway
Developmental Editor: Jessica Demetriou

Obstetrics and Gynecology Clinics (ISSN 0889-8545) is published quarterly by Elsevier Inc., 360 Park Avenue South, New York, NY 10010-1710. Months of issue are March, June, September, and December. Periodicals postage paid at New York, NY, and additional mailing offices. Subscription price per year is $257.00 (US individuals), $431.00 (US institutions), $130.00 (US students), $309.00 (Canadian individuals), $544.00 (Canadian institutions), $191.00 (Canadian students), $376.00 (foreign individuals), $544.00 (foreign institutions), and $191.00 (foreign students). To receive student/resident rate, orders must be accompanied by name of affiliated institution, date of term, and the signature of program/residency coordinator on institution letterhead. Orders will be billed at individual rate until proof of status is received. Foreign air speed delivery is included in all *Clinics* subscription prices. All prices are subject to change without notice. POSTMASTER: Send address changes to *Obstetrics and Gynecology Clinics*, Elsevier Health Sciences Division, Subscription Customer Service, 3251 Riverport Lane, Maryland Heights, MO 63043. **Customer Service: Telephone: 1-800-654-2452 (U.S. and Canada); 314-447-8871 (outside U.S. and Canada). Fax: 314-447-8029. E-mail: journals customerservice-usa@elsevier.com (for print support); journalsonlinesupport-usa@elsevier.com (for online support).**

Reprints. For copies of 100 or more of articles in this publication, please contact the Commercial Reprints Department, Elsevier Inc., 360 Park Avenue South, New York, New York 10010-1710. Tel.: 212-633-3818; Fax: 212-462-1935; E-mail: reprints@elsevier.com.

Obstetrics and Gynecology Clinics of North America is also published in Spanish by McGraw-Hill Interamericana Editores S.A., P.O. Box 5-237, 06500, Mexico; in Portuguese by Reichmann and Affonso Editores, Rio de Janeiro, Brazil; and in Greek by Paschalidis Medical Publications, Athens, Greece.

Obstetrics and Gynecology Clinics of North America is covered in MEDLINE/PubMed (Index Medicus), Excerpta Medica, Current Concepts/Clinical Medicine, Science Citation Index, BIOSIS, CINAHL, and ISI/BIOMED.

Printed and bound by CPI Group (UK) Ltd, Croydon, CR0 4YY

Transferred to Digital Print 2011

GOAL STATEMENT

The goal of *Obstetrics and Gynecology Clinics of North America* is to keep practicing physicians up to date with current clinical practice in OB/GYN by providing timely articles reviewing the state of the art in patient care.

ACCREDITATION

The *Obstetrics and Gynecology Clinics of North America* is planned and implemented in accordance with the Essential Areas and Policies of the Accreditation Council for Continuing Medical Education (ACCME) through the joint sponsorship of the University of Virginia School of Medicine and Elsevier. The University of Virginia School of Medicine is accredited by the ACCME to provide continuing medical education for physicians.

The University of Virginia School of Medicine designates this educational activity for a maximum of 15 *AMA PRA Category 1 Credits*™ for each issue, 60 credits per year. Physicians should only claim credit commensurate with the extent of their participation in the activity.

The American Medical Association has determined that physicians not licensed in the US who participate in this CME activity are eligible for a maximum of 15 *AMA PRA Category 1 Credits*™ for each issue, 60 credits per year.

Category 1 credit can be earned by reading the text material, taking the CME examination online at http://www.theclinics.com/home/cme, and completing the evaluation. After taking the test, you will be required to review any and all incorrect answers. Following completion of the test and evaluation, your credit will be awarded and you may print your certificate.

FACULTY DISCLOSURE/CONFLICT OF INTEREST

The University of Virginia School of Medicine, as an ACCME accredited provider, endorses and strives to comply with the Accreditation Council for Continuing Medical Education (ACCME) Standards of Commercial Support, Commonwealth of Virginia statutes, University of Virginia policies and procedures, and associated federal and private regulations and guidelines on the need for disclosure and monitoring of proprietary and financial interests that may affect the scientific integrity and balance of content delivered in continuing medical education activities under our auspices.

The University of Virginia School of Medicine requires that all CME activities accredited through this institution be developed independently and be scientifically rigorous, balanced and objective in the presentation/discussion of its content, theories and practices.

All authors/editors participating in an accredited CME activity are expected to disclose to the readers relevant financial relationships with commercial entities occurring within the past 12 months (such as grants or research support, employee, consultant, stock holder, member of speakers bureau, etc.). The University of Virginia School of Medicine will employ appropriate mechanisms to resolve potential conflicts of interest to maintain the standards of fair and balanced education to the reader. Questions about specific strategies can be directed to the Office of Continuing Medical Education, University of Virginia School of Medicine, Charlottesville, Virginia.

The faculty and staff of the University of Virginia Office of Continuing Medical Education have no financial affiliations to disclose.

The authors/editors listed below have identified no professional or financial affiliations for themselves or their spouse/partner:
Megan R. Billow, DO; Amber D. Bradshaw, MD; Nichole M. Giannios, DO; Vanessa M. Givens, MD; Carla Holloway (Acquisitions Editor); William W. Hurd, MD, MSc; William Irvin, MD (Test Author); Gary H. Lipscomb, MD; Stephanie D. Pickett, MD; Katherine J. Rodewald, MD; Howard T. Sharp, MD (Guest Editor); David E. Soper, MD; Carolyn Swensen, MD; and Willis H. Wagner, MD.

The authors/editors listed below identified the following professional or financial affiliations for themselves or their spouse/partner:
Arnold P. Advincula, MD is a consultant for Intuitive Surgical, Cooper Surgical, and Ethicon Endo-Surgery.
Gweneth B. Lazenby, MD is an industry funded research/investigator for GenProbe.
Malcolm G. Munro, MD, FRCS(c) is a consultant for Karl Storz Endoscopy Americas, Ethicon Women's Health and Urology, Bayer Women's Health Care, and AMAG Pharmaceuticals; is on the Advisory Committee/Board of Ethicon Women's Health and Urology; and is an industry funded research/investigator for Bayer Women's Health Care.
William H. Parker, MD is a consultant for Ethicon.
William F. Rayburn, MD, MBA (Consulting Editor) is an industry funded research/investigator and a consultant for Cytokine PharmaSciences.

Disclosure of Discussion of non-FDA approved uses for pharmaceutical products and/or medical devices:

The University of Virginia School of Medicine, as an ACCME provider, requires that all faculty presenters identify and disclose any off-label uses for pharmaceutical and medical device products. The University of Virginia School of Medicine recommends that each physician fully review all the available data on new products or procedures prior to clinical use.

TO ENROLL

To enroll in the Obstetrics and Gynecology Clinics of North America Continuing Medical Education program, call customer service at 1-800-654-2452 or visit us online at www.theclinics.com/home/cme. The CME program is available to subscribers for an additional fee of $180.00

Contributors

CONSULTING EDITOR

WILLIAM F. RAYBURN, MD, MBA
Randolph Seligman Professor and Chair, Department of Obstetrics and Gynecology;
Chief of Staff, University Hospital, University of New Mexico Health Science Center,
Albuquerque, New Mexico

GUEST EDITOR

HOWARD T. SHARP, MD
Associate Professor and Vice Chair for Clinical Affairs, Department of Obstetrics
and Gynecology, University of Utah Health Sciences Center, Salt Lake City, Utah

AUTHORS

ARNOLD P. ADVINCULA, MD
Professor of Obstetrics & Gynecology, University of Central Florida College of Medicine,
Center for Specialized Gynecology, Florida Hospital, Celebration Health, Celebration,
Florida

MEGAN R. BILLOW, DO
Obstetrics and Gynecology Resident Physician, University Hospitals Case Medical
Center, Cleveland, Ohio

AMBER D. BRADSHAW, MD
Fellow in Minimally Invasive Surgery, University of Central Florida College of Medicine,
Center for Specialized Gynecology, Florida Hospital, Celebration Health, Celebration,
Florida

NICHOLE M. GIANNIOS, DO
Reproductive Endocrinology and Infertility Fellow, Department of Obstetrics and
Gynecology, University Hospitals Case Medical Center, Cleveland, Ohio

VANESSA M. GIVENS, MD
Associate Professor, Section of Obstetrics and Gynecology, Department of Family
Medicine, University of Tennessee Health Science Center, Memphis, Tennessee

WILLIAM W. HURD, MD, MSc
Lilian Hanna Baldwin Endowed Chair in Gynecology and Obstetrics; Director, Division
of Reproductive Endocrinology and Infertility, Department of Obstetrics and Gynecology,
University Hospitals Case Medical Center; Professor of Reproductive Biology, Case
Western Reserve University School of Medicine, Cleveland, Ohio

GWENETH B. LAZENBY, MD
Clinical Instructor and Reproductive Infectious Diseases Fellow, Department of Obstetrics
and Gynecology, Medical University of South Carolina, Charleston, South Carolina

GARY H. LIPSCOMB, MD
Professor, Section of Obstetrics and Gynecology, Department of Family Medicine,
University of Tennessee Health Science Center, Memphis, Tennessee

MALCOLM G. MUNRO, MD, FACOG, FRCS(c)
Professor, Department of Obstetrics and Gynecology, David Geffen School of Medicine
at University of California Los Angeles; Director of Gynecologic Services, Department
of Obstetrics and Gynecology, Kaiser-Permanente, Los Angeles Medical Center,
Los Angeles, California

WILLIAM H. PARKER, MD
Clinical Professor, Department of Obstetrics and Gynecology, University of California
Los Angeles School of Medicine, Los Angeles; Saint John's Health Center, Santa Monica,
California

STEPHANIE D. PICKETT, MD
Obstetrics and Gynecology Resident Physician, University Hospitals Case Medical
Center, Cleveland, Ohio

KATHERINE J. RODEWALD, MD
Obstetrics and Gynecology Resident Physician, University Hospitals Case Medical
Center, Cleveland, Ohio

HOWARD T. SHARP, MD
Associate Professor and Vice Chair for Clinical Affairs, Department of Obstetrics and
Gynecology, University of Utah Health Sciences Center, Salt Lake City, Utah

DAVID E. SOPER, MD
Professor of Obstetrics and Gynecology, Department of Obstetrics and Gynecology,
Medical University of South Carolina, Charleston, South Carolina

CAROLYN SWENSON, MD
Resident Physician, Department of Obstetrics and Gynecology, University of Utah Health
Sciences Center, Salt Lake City, Utah

WILLIS H. WAGNER, MD
Medical Director, Vascular Laboratory, Saint John's Health Center, Santa Monica,
California

Contents

Electrosurgery is used on a daily basis in the operating room, but it remains poorly understood by those using it. In addition, the physics of electrosurgery are far more complicated than those of laser. Common belief notwithstanding, electrosurgery has an enormous capacity for patient injury if used incorrectly, even though technology has markedly reduced the likelihood of patient or surgeon injuries. This article is intended to educate the clinician regarding the basis of electrosurgery and provide an explanation on how injuries may occur as well as how they may be prevented.

Surgical site Infections (SSIs) have a significant effect on patient care and medical costs. This article outlines the risks that lead to SSIs and the preventive measures, including antimicrobial prophylaxis, which decrease the incidence of infection. This article also reviews the diagnosis and treatment of gynecologic SSIs.

Major vessel injuries during laparoscopy most commonly occur during insertion of Veress needle and port trocars through the abdominal wall. This article reviews methods for avoiding major vessel injury while gaining laparoscopic access, including anatomic relationships of abdominal wall landmarks to the major retroperitoneal vessels. Methods for periumbilical placement of the Veress needle and primary trocar are reviewed in terms of direction and angle of insertion, and alternative methods and locations are discussed. Methods for secondary port placement are reviewed in terms of direction, depth, and speed of placement.

Adverse events associated with hysteroscopic procedures are in general rare, but, with increasing operative complexity, it is now apparent that

they are experienced more often. A spectrum of complications exist ranging from those that relate to generic components of procedures such as
patient positioning and anesthesia and analgesia, to a number that are
specific to intraluminal endoscopic surgery (perforation and injuries to surrounding structures and blood vessels). The response of premenopausal
women to excessive absorption of nonionic fluids deserves special attention. There is also an increasing awareness of uncommon but problematic
sequelae related to the use of monopolar uterine resectoscopes that involve thermal injury to the vulva and vagina. The uterus that has previously
undergone hysteroscopic surgery can behave in unusual ways, at least in
premenopausal women who experience menstruation or who become
pregnant. Better understanding of the mechanisms involved in these adverse events, as well as the use or development of several devices, have
collectively provided the opportunity to perform hysteroscopic and resectoscopic surgery in a manner that minimizes risk to the patient.

Surgical blood loss of more than 1000 mL or blood loss that requires
a blood transfusion usually defines intraoperative hemorrhage. Intraoperative hemorrhage has been reported in 1% to 2% of hysterectomy studies.
Preoperative evaluation of the patient can aid surgical planning to help prevent intraoperative hemorrhage or prepare for the management of hemorrhage, should it occur. To this effect, the medical and medication history
and use of alternative medication must be gathered. This article discusses
the methods of preoperative management of anemia, including use of iron,
recombinant erythropoietin, and gonadotropin-releasing hormone agonists. The authors have also reviewed the methods of intraoperative and
postoperative management of bleeding.

Complications may occur during laparoscopic surgery, even with a skilled
surgeon and under ideal circumstances; human error is inevitable. Videotaped procedures from malpractice cases are evaluated to ascertain potential contributing cognitive factors, systems errors, equipment issues,
and surgeon training. Situation awareness and principles derived from aviation crew resource management may be adapted to help avoid systems
error. The current process of surgical training may need to be reconsidered.

The development of a postoperative neuropathy is a rare complication that
can be devastating to the patient. Most cases of postoperative neuropathy
are caused by improper patient positioning and the incorrect placement of
surgical retractors. This article presents the nerves that are at greatest risk
of injury during gynecologic surgery through a series of vignettes. Suggestions for protection of each nerve are provided.

Hollow Viscus Injury During Surgery   461

Howard T. Sharp and Carolyn Swenson

Reproductive tract surgery carries a risk of injury to the bladder, ureter, and gastrointestinal (GI) tract. This is due to several factors including close surgical proximity of these organs, disease processes that can distort anatomy, delayed mechanical and energy effects, and the inability to directly visualize organ surfaces. The purpose of this article is to review strategies to prevent, recognize, and repair injury to the GI and urinary tract during gynecologic surgery.

Index   469

RELATED INTEREST

Obstetrics and Gynecology Clinics of North America March 2008 (Vol. 35, Issue 1)
Patient Safety in Obstetrics and Gynecology: Improving Outcomes, Reducing Risks
Paul A. Gluck, MD, *Guest Editor*
www.obgyn.theclinics.com

THE CLINICS ARE NOW AVAILABLE ONLINE!

Access your subscription at:
www.theclinics.com

Foreword

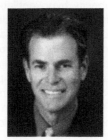

William F. Rayburn, MD, MBA
Consulting Editor

A patient's operative care should be planned with attention to detail and awareness of potential complications. This issue, guest edited by Dr Howard Sharp, pertains to the prevention and management of complications from gynecologic surgery. Major objectives are to restore the patient's physiologic and psychologic health. The operating room presents the possibility for immediate or delayed errors. Adverse surgical events are relatively infrequent compared with other types of medical errors, although these problems often receive increased attention.

This distinguished group of authors comes from academic health centers. Graduate medical education requires full supervision and assistance by qualified and experienced gynecologists. It is up to the clinical judgment of the supervising surgeon to allow increasing operative responsibilities for trainees based on their experience, skill, and level of training. Expanding training by using surgical simulators and virtual training techniques helps better prepare trainees before entering the operating suite.

The American College of Obstetricians and Gynecologists' Committee Opinion Number 328 states that "ensuring patient safety in the operating room begins before she enters the operative suite and includes attention to all applicable types of preventable medical errors (including, for example, medication errors) but surgical errors are unique to this environment." A single error may lead to a grave patient injury even with the most vigilant supervision. Communication issues, unique terminology, and special instruments must be understood and shared by all members of the team.

There is a complication rate for every operation. Patients need to understand the risks and benefits of the procedure, as well as any alternatives, before a gynecologist initiates any therapy. Informed consent is a discussion, not simply a form. This issue describes the management of certain complications of gynecologic surgery, which include electrosurgical energy-related injury, excess hemorrhage, major vessel injury and venous thromboembolism, and urinary tract and bowel injuries. In the elderly and obese patients, respiratory insufficiency is an especially common postoperative problem.

Obstet Gynecol Clin N Am 37 (2010) xi–xii
doi:10.1016/j.ogc.2010.06.002
0889-8545/10/$ – see front matter © 2010 Elsevier Inc. All rights reserved.

obgyn.theclinics.com

Obesity is becoming more prevalent in our surgical patients and represents a much higher risk for surgical complications. The occurrence of comorbidities, including diabetes, hypertension, coronary artery disease, sleep apnea, obesity hypoventilation syndrome, and osteoarthritis of the knees and hips, are more frequent. These underlying alterations in physiology result in increased surgical risks of cardiac failure, deep venous and pulmonary emboli, aspiration, wound infection and dehiscence, postoperative neuropathy, and misdiagnosed intra-abdominal catastrophe.

It is our desire that this issue inspires attention to a vast array of operative complications. On behalf of Dr Sharp and his excellent team of knowledgeable contributors, I hope that the practical information provided herein will aid in the implementation of evidence-based and well-planned approaches to preventing and managing complications from gynecologic surgery.

William F. Rayburn, MD, MBA
Department of Obstetrics and Gynecology
University of New Mexico School of Medicine
MSC10 5580, 1 University of New Mexico, Albuquerque
NM 87131-0001, USA

E-mail address:
wrayburn@salud.unm.edu

Preface
Surgical Complications

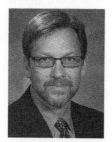

Howard T. Sharp, MD
Guest Editor

It is more enjoyable to read about complications than to manage them. Surgical complications are challenging for several reasons. It is difficult to watch patients and their families suffer. Although some complications are minor setbacks that resolve over time, some lead to longstanding disability. As surgeons, we sometimes doubt ourselves in the wake of a complication and lose confidence in our abilities. In some cases, surgeons avoid surgery or practice heightened defensive surgery, rendering them surgically dysfunctional. We should ask ourselves, "Is there something I should have done differently?" "Could this have been avoided?" and "Should I have recognized something earlier?" These are questions I ask each week at our institution's morbidity and mortality conference.

One of my favorite surgical mentors, the great, late Gary Johnson, MD, would lament, "If you don't want surgical complications, don't do surgery." He had figured out that complications happen. I do not know that he was any more comfortable with complications than I, but he recognized an important truth: there is a complication rate for each surgery performed. Are there ways to reduce complication rates? I think so. Can all complications be eliminated? I think not.

It has always sounded a bit ridiculous to me when someone says, "He or she has the hands of a surgeon," as if the hands have so much to do with being a good surgeon. Having a steady hand and knowing the patient and how to perform surgery are given basic prerequisites for taking a patient to the operating room. But there is much more to being a good surgeon. Surgeons must know anatomy and anatomic variation, be familiar with surgical instrumentation and its technology, have situational awareness, and be ever vigilant to recognize risks for complications preoperatively, intraoperatively, and postoperatively. Some have said it is good to have a little healthy paranoia. The reason for vigilance is the recurrent theme of early recognition and management of complications associated with better outcomes. If there were anything

Obstet Gynecol Clin N Am 37 (2010) xiii–xiv
doi:10.1016/j.ogc.2010.05.005
0889-8545/10/$ – see front matter
obgyn.theclinics.com

to stress in the volume, it is that avoiding complications is much more than just having "good hands." It is my sincere hope that the words of these fine authors will allow the readers to avoid and manage complications to the best of their ability.

Howard T. Sharp, MD
Department of Obstetrics and Gynecology
University of Utah Health Sciences Center
Room 2B-200, 1900 East, 30 North
Salt Lake City, UT 84132, USA

E-mail address:
howard.sharp@hsc.utah.edu

Preventing Electrosurgical Energy–Related Injuries

Gary H. Lipscomb, MD*, Vanessa M. Givens, MD

KEYWORDS

- Electrosurgery • Electrode • Cut current • Coagulation current

In 1928, Cushing[1] reported a series of 500 neurosurgical procedures on the brain in which bleeding was controlled by an electrosurgical unit designed by W.T. Bovie. Since that time, the "Bovie" has become an instrument familiar to every gynecologic surgeon. Most gynecologic surgeons would consider it a much simpler and safer instrument than the carbon-dioxide or KTP laser or the argon beam coagulator. This belief is reinforced by the fact that even weekend introductory laser courses present a thorough review of laser physics, whereas lectures on electrosurgery are uncommon even in advanced operative gynecology courses. Common belief notwithstanding, electrosurgery has an enormous capacity for patient injury if used incorrectly. In addition, the physics of electrosurgery are far more complicated than those of laser. This article reviews the principles of electrosurgery and the mechanisms of electrosurgical injury and discusses the methods of prevention of these injuries.

ELECTROPHYSICS

Although a detailed description of electrophysics is beyond the scope of this article, it is necessary to review some of the basic principles of electrosurgery to understand why patient injuries occur. The most fundamental principles of electrosurgery are that electricity always seeks the ground and the path of least resistance. These 2 principles are straightforward and even intuitive. However, most of the other principles of electrosurgery are not so easily understood. Because most physicians find electrophysics confusing, it is often easier to relate many of the terms to those of hydraulics, which are more familiar. Just as a certain amount of water flows through a garden hose, electric energy consists of a flow of negatively charged particles called electrons. This flow of electrons is referred to as current. Electric current is described by

---

Section of Obstetrics and Gynecology, Department of Family Medicine, University of Tennessee Health Science Center, 1301 Primacy Parkway, Memphis, TN 38119, USA
* Corresponding author.
E-mail address: garyhlipscomb@gmail.com

Obstet Gynecol Clin N Am 37 (2010) 369–377
doi:10.1016/j.ogc.2010.05.007
0889-8545/10/$ – see front matter © 2010 Elsevier Inc. All rights reserved.

obgyn.theclinics.com

several interrelated terms.[2] First, current is measured by the number of electrons flowing per second. A flow of 6.24×10^{18} electrons (1 coulomb [C]) per second is referred to as 1 A. This is analogous to a stream of water in which the flow is measured in gallons per minute. Volt is the unit of force that drives the electron flow against resistance, and 1 V drives 1 A of current through a specified resistance. The volt is similar to water in a hose under a force of so many pounds per square inch. As with water in a hose, the higher the water pressure the greater the potential for leaks to occur. Similarly, in the case of electricity, the higher the voltage the greater the possibility of unwanted stray current. The difficulty that a substance presents to the flow of current is known as resistance and is sometimes referred to as impedance (I). Resistance is measured in ohm. The power of current, measured in watts, is the amount of work produced by the electron flow. Again using the water analogy, power is equivalent to the work in horsepower produced by a stream of water as it turns a waterwheel. Power can also be related to the heat output and is often measured in British thermal unit. **Table 1** shows the relationship between these terms.

All variables in electrosurgery are closely interrelated such that a change in one variable leads to changes in the others. Using the analogy of water flowing through a pipe, it is probably intuitive that if the resistance to flow is increased by decreasing the diameter of the pipe, the pressure forcing the water through the pipe must be increased to maintain the previous flow rate. Similar events occur with electrosurgery. If the tissue resistance increases, voltage must also be increased to maintain a constant power. This interrelationship is known as Ohm's law, which states that the current in an electric circuit is directly proportional to the voltage and inversely proportional to the resistance.

An electric current consists of either a direct or an alternating current. Direct current is the same current produced by batteries, whereas alternating current is the same current that is used at home. **Fig. 1** illustrates the pattern generated on an oscilloscope by the 2 different types of currents. Direct current produces a flow of electrons from one electric pole to another of opposite charge. The flow of current is unidirectional and continuous. One pole is always negatively charged, and the other is always positively charged. Direct current is not normally used in electrosurgery.

Unlike direct current in which the poles are always the same charge, in alternating current the poles reverse polarity periodically. As a result, alternating current alternates the direction of electron flow, first flowing in one direction then reversing flow. The rate at which the polarity reverses is described in cycles per second and is referred to as the frequency of the cycle. One cycle per second is 1 Hz. Electric current used at home is supplied as alternating current at 60 Hz. Voltage of alternating current is normally measured either from zero baseline to maximum (peak voltage) or from the maximum in one direction to the maximum in the other (peak-to-peak voltage). Average or mean voltage when describing alternating current is meaningless because the positive voltage in one cycle is negated by the identical negative voltage in the

Table 1		
Equivalent terms for electricity and hydraulics		
Term	**Unit**	**Hydraulic Equivalent**
Current	Ampere	Gallons per minute
Voltage	Volt	Pounds per square inch
Impedance	Ohm	Resistance
Power	Watt	Horsepower

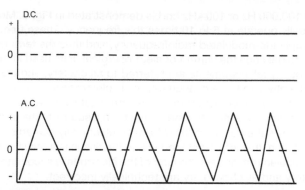

Fig. 1. Direct and alternating current. AC, alternating current; DC, direct current.

same cycle. Thus the average voltage of the current would be zero. To avoid this problem, the average peak voltage is described using a standard statistical measure that describes the magnitude using the square root of the mean of the squares of the values or the root-mean-square (RMS) value. The RMS of household current is 120 V. **Fig. 2** illustrates these terms as illustrated with household current.

EFFECTS

Why do patients do not have muscle contraction or pain when undergoing electrosurgical procedures? Common answers are that the patient is grounded or under anesthesia. A patient undergoing a loop electrosurgical excision procedure is not under anesthesia but does not have muscle contraction. Few people would want to ground themselves by pouring water on the floor and then stick their finger in a light socket. Why then patients do not experience nerve and muscle excitation?

Normally, when a direct electric current is applied to a tissue, the positively and negatively charged particles in the cells migrate to the oppositely charged poles and the cell membranes undergo depolarization resulting in muscle contraction and nerve stimulation. This is known as the Faraday effect. With alternating current, the electric poles reverse with each cycle. If the frequency becomes high enough, there is insufficient time between cycles for the charged ions to migrate before the poles reverse. At this point, nerve and muscle depolarization does not occur. This effect occurs at

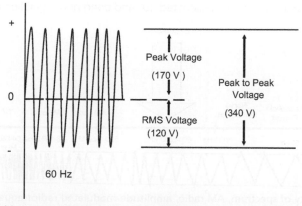

Fig. 2. Household current (voltage, cycle, and RMS).

approximately 100,000 Hz or 100 kHz and is demonstrated in **Fig. 3**. Most electrosurgical units actually operate at 5 to 10 times this frequency. These frequencies are in the range of amplitude-modulated radiofrequency, and thus the term radiofrequency current is used to describe the current of electrosurgical units used in medicine.

Often, electrosurgical instruments are referred to as cautery, and the term electrocautery is frequently used interchangeably with electrocoagulation to indicate the coagulation of tissue with electric current. The term cautery is derived from the Greek "kauterion" or hot iron. A cautery transfers heat from a source to the tissue, and therefore electrocautery is the transfer of heat from an electrically heated source to tissue. In electrocoagulation, the heat developed within the tissue is a result of the resistance to the passage of electron, and any heating of the electrode is secondary to this. Thus, the terms cautery and electrocautery are technically incorrect.

MONOPOLAR AND BIPOLAR CURRENTS

Electrosurgery can be divided into monopolar or bipolar depending on the number of electric poles at the site of application. In reality, all electric devices require 2 poles to complete an electric current. With unipolar current, the Bovie tip is one pole, whereas the second pole is the grounding pad. With bipolar current, both poles are part of the tip of the instrument. The main difference between the 2 types of current is the distance between the poles. Because the human body is a relatively poor conductor of electric current, a relatively high power output is needed to overcome the long distance between the poles in unipolar electrosurgery. With bipolar instruments, the electrodes are only millimeters apart. Because a high-power current would destroy the instrument, the power output of bipolar instruments is one-third to one-tenth that of unipolar systems. The relatively low power of bipolar systems is insufficient to generate the current densities that are needed to cut tissue, and thus these systems can only desiccate the tissue. Because of the constant inflow of electrons, a nonmodulated cutting waveform produces a more uniform desiccation than a modulated coagulation current. Coagulation current tends to produce a rapid superficial desiccation that impedes further electron flow into the center. For this reason, bipolar electrosurgical generators designed for tubal sterilization produce only cut current because the use of coagulation current has been associated with higher failure rates.

CUT AND COAGULATION CURRENTS

Electrosurgical generators produce 2 primary types of alternating current, which have, through common usage, been designated cut and coag or coagulation currents. But,

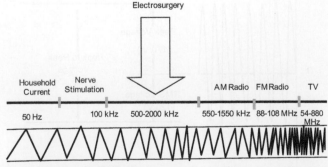

Fig. 3. Frequency of spectrum. AM radio, amplitude-modulated radiofrequency; FM radio, frequency-modulated radiofrequency.

these labels are misleading because they do not necessarily produce the tissue effects that are associated with the terms cut and coagulation. In fact, cut current can coagulate and coag current can cut, but cut current is often the most appropriate current to use for tissue coagulation. Cut current is more accurately designated as nonmodulated or undamped current, and coag current is designated as modulated or damped current. Nonmodulated cut current is characterized by a continuous uninterrupted flow of electrons. Modulated coag or damped current consists of a burst of alternating current interrupted by intervals of no current flow. Fully modulated current has no current flow for more than 95% of each cycle. **Fig. 4** illustrates the 2 types of currents. At identical power levels, there is less current flow per time interval with modulated current than with nonmodulated current. Because power (W) = volts (V) × current flow (I), the peak-to-peak voltage of modulated current must be greater to produce the same power of nonmodulated current. More simply, for the same wattage, coag current has a much higher voltage than cut current. As previously noted, higher voltages are more likely to produce unwanted effects and injuries than lower voltages. In more simple terms, for the same power levels, cut current is the safer modality.

ELECTROSURGICAL CUTTING

Electrosurgical cutting occurs when the intracellular temperature increases high and fast enough to cause the explosive vaporization of water. Electrosurgical cutting occurs only under extremely high current densities that exist when the current is confined to arcs traveling between the electrode and tissue (**Fig. 5**). Cutting is facilitated by conditions that encourage the formation of these arcs. Arcs are further enhanced by the steam envelope formed around the electrode by the vaporization of cellular water. A continuous current (nonmodulated or cut current) is necessary to maintain this vapor barrier. Efficient cutting requires the electrode to be moved slowly but continuously through the tissue. Moving too quickly collapses the steam barrier and places the electrode in contact with tissue. Because the cross-sectional area of the electrode is greater than that of the arc, the current density decreases than that needed for cutting, and the electrode stalls until the steam barrier is regained. Therefore, if tissue cutting is desired, the electrode should be activated before touching the tissue and moved slowly to avoid dragging.

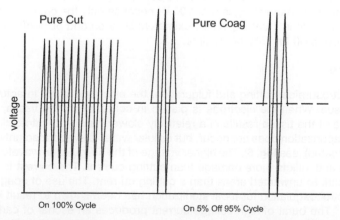

Fig. 4. Cut versus coag current.

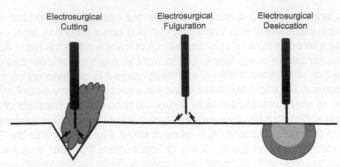

Fig. 5. Cutting, fulguration, and desiccation.

SPRAY COAGULATION (FULGURATION)

Spray coagulation or fulguration is different from electrosurgical cutting. In fulguration, high-voltage, interrupted current (modulated or coag current) is required. The higher voltages of modulated current compared with those of nonmodulated current allow arcs to form to the tissue in the absence of a vapor barrier (see **Fig. 5**). Because the coagulation waveform is highly interrupted, any steam barrier formed collapses before the next cycle. The result is that the arcs strike a wider area of tissue in a random fashion. Much like lightning, it is never said to strike twice in the same spot. With the coagulation waveform, there is less-rapid heating of tissue because the pause allows heat to be dissipated to other cells. The end result is more cell heating and dehydration, with more charring than that occurring with electrosurgical cutting. However, the effect is superficial.

BLENDED CURRENT

Blended current is not, as is frequently misbelieved, a blend of cut and coag currents, but it actually refers to a blending of effects. Use of blended current helps to cut tissue while obtaining some degree of coagulation but avoiding the thicker eschar associated with cutting in the full coag mode. Blended current is obtained by modulating the normal cut current so that the cycle is off for a percentage of time less than that obtained in the full coag mode. The coag setting on the generator is irrelevant. Therefore, if a setting of blend 1 is selected with a cut setting of 40 W, the effect will be the same whether the coag setting is 0 or 100 W because only the cut current is modulated. Typically, blend 1 setting is approximately 50% on and 50% off. Blend 3 has the current cycle off for 75% of the time.

DESICCATION

In both electrosurgical cutting and fulguration, the electrode is not in actual contact with the tissue. When the electrode is placed in contact with the tissue, the larger surface area of the tissue results in a relatively slower heating of intracellular water. Explosive vaporization does not occur, but cellular water is evaporated until the tissue is dry (desiccated) (see **Fig. 5**). The higher voltage of the coagulation waveform is more penetrating and inflicts more damage than cutting current. The current is also more prone to spark to unwanted areas than a cutting current. The use of coag current in bipolar electrocoagulation for tubal sterilization has been shown to result in a higher failure rate.[3] The burst of high-voltage current produces an eschar of carbon at the surface of the tube. The eschar inhibits penetration of the current into the interior of the tube and may result in inadequate coagulation, leaving a viable tubal lumen. The slower crock-pot desiccation produced with cutting current produces a more complete coagulation.

Coaptive coagulation is another form of desiccation that involves clamping a bleeding vessel with a conductive clamp and applying current to the clamp to produce a collagen weld of the vessel. Because of previously mentioned factors, cutting current is usually the most appropriate current for this purpose, which is opposite to the belief of most surgeons. As noted later in this article, use of coag current in this setting is much more likely to lead to a surgeon being zapped or burned.

As with lasers, the effect of electric current on tissue depends on the amount of power applied per square centimeter of surface area multiplied by time. In monopolar mode, the active electrode is usually small, whereas the ground electrode is relatively larger. The same amount of current flows out of the ground pad as enters from the active electrode. However, because the current is dispersed over a wide area, no tissue damage occurs. Severe burns can occur if the pad becomes detached except for a small area. The tissue effect at the pad then approaches that encountered at the active electrode. Similarly, the use of a needle-tip electrode results in high current densities that cuts the tissue with minimum lateral thermal damage, whereas a broader-blade electrode produces more thermal tissue damage.

INJURIES WITH ELECTROSURGERY

Unintended burns may occur in several ways during electrosurgery.[4] Burns may occur at the active electrode as a result of direct coupling, away from the active electrode as a result of capacitance coupling, or from alternate path burn.

Perhaps the most common type of electrosurgical injury results from direct application of current to tissue away from the active electrode itself (direct coupling). The most easily understood example of this type of injury is when another metal object such as a probe is touched by the active electrode. The current is conducted through the probe resulting in injury to the tissue where the probe touches. Injury may also occur if a metal retractor is touched by a hemostat that is being energized to coagulate a bleeding patient. The contact may go unnoticed and unrecognized until the following day when a full-thickness burn is noted on the skin 1 or 2 in away from the incision, seeming far away from the region where electrosurgery was done. This burnt site is in reality an area where the retractor was resting on the skin. Another example of this type of injury occurs when a defect in insulation allows the current to flow from the defect into the adjacent tissue.

Direct coupling is best avoided by situational awareness of where the active electrode is at all times when the electrode is being energized. Particular care should be exercised anytime the active electrode is energized near another metal object. Insulation failure is more difficult to avoid. Frequent inspection of reusable insulated instruments may detect insulation flaws before injury occurs. Use of disposable instruments reduces the chance of repetitive use resulting in damage to insulation that may then result in patient injuries. There are also conductive sheaths available that when placed over the instrument monitor for stray current and shut down the generator if such current is detected.

Alternate Path Burns

The original Bovie electrosurgical unit was a grounded instrument. As such, current eventually flows into an electron sink or ground, which originally was the earth. As previously noted, electricity always seeks the path of least resistance to ground. In grounded systems, if there is impedance to the flow of electrons to the ground via the intended path, other conductive objects may become the path of least resistance. The other objects could be the metal table in an operating room or the electrocardiogram (ECG) leads on the patient. Because of the small size of the ECG leads, deep burns may occur if current is diverted through them.

The likelihood of alternate site burns was considerably reduced by the introduction of isolated electrosurgical generators in 1972. These generators are no longer connected to a true ground. If a reduction in current flow back to the generator is detected, the generator shuts down. This mode of action markedly reduces the probability of alternate site injuries. Another consequence of this technology is that the ground pads themselves have been eliminated. The correct term for the pads that are available today is patient return electrode.

Patient Electrode Burn

In monopolar electrosurgery, the current travels through the patient between 2 active electrodes. Normally, no effect is seen at the return electrode because of its larger surface area. If for some reason the return electrode becomes detached or has been improperly placed, patient injury may occur. Because the return electrode is typically out of direct sight, a large, deep, full-thickness burn may occur without the surgeon's knowledge.

The introduction of return electrode monitoring (REM) technology has essentially eliminated this type of patient injury. In REM, the return electrode is divided into 2 electrodes that are electrically connected to each other by the patient's skin. A low-intensity current is constantly passed between the 2 electrodes. If this current is not detected because the electrode has become detached or if the surface temperature increases by more than 2°C, the generator deactivates.

Capacitance Coupling

When unidirectional electric current travels through a conductor, an electromagnetic field is generated around the conductor. This field can generate a secondary current in nearby conductors, such as a metal trocar. The amount of current generated is determined by multiple factors. Capacitance coupling is increased with increasing voltage. Because coag current is associated with higher voltage it is more likely to result in a capacitance effect. Open circuit activation (current activation without touching tissue) also markedly increases voltage and thus the risk of capacitance. The use of cutting current and limiting the open circuit activation decreases the risk.

Capacitive coupling can produce sufficient current to cause an injury under several conditions. The most common is when a metal cannula is used with a plastic tissue anchor. Current can be induced on the metal cannula, but return of current via the abdominal wall is prevented by the plastic anchor. Up to 70% of the originally applied current may be inducted in some circumstances. If this current is not conducted away by the abdominal wall, arcing from the trocar to adjacent tissue may occur. The area where arcing occurs is frequently out of the visual field of the surgeon and may result in significant injuries. Thus the old adage, "use all metal or all plastic trocars."

As previously noted, the use of conductive sheaths can conduct stray current from the surgical site as well as monitor the total amount of current present before delivering it to the return electrode.

Surgeon Burns

Surgeons may suffer burns from the use of electrosurgical units.[5] Burns may occur from faulty insulation or contact with the active electrode. The cause of these injuries is readily apparent to most clinicians. An injury that is poorly understood by most surgeons is the burn occurring when zapping a hemostat to coagulate a bleeding vessel. This type of coagulation is known as coaptive coagulation. It is commonly believed that coaptive coagulation results from a preexisting hole in the surgical glove; however, surgical gloves offer minimal insulation to electrosurgical current. In reality, the current results in a breakdown of the glove material, that is, it blows a hole in the glove.

There are 4 conditions that increase the likelihood of hemostat burns:

1. The use of coag current with its associated higher voltage is much more likely to result in surgeon burns than the more appropriate cut current.
2. In anticipation of a possible burn, surgeons often instinctively hold the hemostat gingerly resulting in a small surface area between the hemostat and the hand. Similar to the way by which the return electrode's large surface area does not result in a patient burn, a broad grip of the hemostat reduces the likelihood of surgeon burns.
3. The use of open activation circuit producing arcing to the hemostat results in the highest voltage as the generator tries to complete the circuit. Touching the hemostat before activation produces much-lower voltage and less potential for glove failure.
4. Because modern electrosurgical units are not grounded, the surgeon has to become part of the circuit to produce a hemostat burn. Contact with the patient or metal retractors with the hand not grasping the hemostat allows the surgeon to be part of the circuit. Lifting the hand off the patient or releasing the retractors isolates the surgeon and prevents burns from occurring.

SUMMARY

Electrosurgery is used on a daily basis in the operating room, but it remains poorly understood by those using it. Although technology has markedly reduced the likelihood of patient or surgeon injuries, the potential for serious injuries still exists. This article is intended to educate the clinician regarding the basis of electrosurgery and provide an explanation on how injuries may occur as well as how they may be prevented.

REFERENCES

1. Cushing H. Electrosurgery as an aid to the removal of intracranial tumors. Surg Gynecol Obstet 1928;47:751–4.
2. Hulka JF, Reich H. Power: electricity and laser. In: Textbook of laparoscopy. Philadelphia: WB Saunders; 1994. p. 23–46.
3. Engel T, Harris FW. The electric dynamics of laparoscopic sterilization. J Reprod Med 1975;15:33–42.
4. Luciano AA, Soderstrom RM, Martin DM. Essential principles of electrosurgery in operative laparoscopy. J Am Assoc Gynecol Laparosc 1994;1:189–95.
5. Odel RC. Biophysics of electrical energy. In: Soderstrom RM, editor. Operative laparoscopy: the masters' technique. New York: Raven Press; 1993. p. 35–44.

Prevention, Diagnosis, and Treatment of Gynecologic Surgical Site Infections

Gweneth B. Lazenby, MD, David E. Soper, MD*

KEYWORDS

• Surgical site infections • Wound infections
• Antibiotic prophylaxis

Surgical site infections (SSIs) are the most common nosocomial infections encountered during inpatient hospitalization. Approximately two-thirds of these infections involve superficial incisions, and the remaining involve the deeper tissues and organ spaces. SSIs have a significant effect on health care costs by prolonging hospitalization, requiring additional medications, and potentially additional procedures.[1–3] This article reviews the pathophysiology, risk factors, prevention strategies, diagnosis, and treatment of postoperative gynecologic surgical infections.

PATHOPHYSIOLOGY AND MICROBIOLOGY

SSIs are initiated at the time of surgery by endogenous flora of the skin or vagina contaminating the wound. A foreign body, such as suture, decreases the number of organisms necessary for the development of SSI. Most endogenous skin flora are composed of aerobic gram-positive cocci.[4] The most frequent organisms isolated from SSIs of abdominal incisions are *Staphylococcus aureus*, coagulase-negative staphylococci, *Enterococcus* spp, and *Escherichia coli*. During gynecologic procedures, potential pathogenic microorganisms may come from the skin or ascend from the vagina and endocervix to the operative sites, which include abdominal incision, upper genital tract and/or vaginal cuff. Gynecologic SSIs are more likely to be infected with gram-negative bacilli, enterococci, group B streptococci, and anaerobes as a result of incisions involving the vagina, and perineum.[5,6] Postoperative pelvic abscesses are commonly associated with anaerobes.[6,7] Bacterial vaginosis alters

Department of Obstetrics and Gynecology, Medical University of South Carolina, 96 Jonathon Lucas Street, Suite 634 MSC 619, Charleston, SC 29425, USA
* Corresponding author.
E-mail address: soperde@musc.edu

Obstet Gynecol Clin N Am 37 (2010) 379–386
doi:10.1016/j.ogc.2010.05.001
0889-8545/10/$ – see front matter © 2010 Elsevier Inc. All rights reserved.

the vaginal flora to increase the concentration of anaerobes by 1000- to 10,000-fold. This increase in anaerobes is an important risk factor in the development of postoperative pelvic infection, especially vaginal cuff cellulitis.[8,9] In recent years, methicillin-resistant S aureus (MRSA) has played a larger role in SSIs.[1]

RISK FACTORS

Risk factors for SSIs include diabetes, tobacco abuse, systemic steroid use, surgical site irradiation, poor nutrition, obesity, prolonged perioperative stay, and transfusion of blood products.[1,7,10] Preoperative vaginitis due to bacterial vaginosis or Trichomonas vaginalis is associated with increased risk of posthysterectomy cuff cellulitis.[2,8] Women should be screened for vaginitis and treated before surgery to decrease this risk.[9] Cervical infection with Chlamydia trachomatis, Neisseria gonorrhoeae, and mycoplasmas can lead to ascending infection during transcervical procedures. Preoperative screening for cervicitis is recommended in women at risk for sexually transmitted infections. Surgical factors associated with SSIs include prolonged surgery duration, excessive blood loss, hypothermia, hair removal by shaving, and the use of surgical drains.[1,10–12] Patients undergoing abdominal hysterectomy are more likely to experience febrile morbidity than those who undergo vaginal hysterectomy.[12]

Nasal carriage of S aureus and MRSA has been associated with an increased risk of SSIs after certain operations; specifically, cardiothoracic, neurosurgical, and orthopedic surgeries.[10] In these cases, nasal application of mupirocin ointment before surgery has been shown to decrease the microbial burden.[4,13] There are no data regarding the effect of S aureus and MRSA decolonization before gynecologic surgeries.

PREVENTION

Surgical practices that decrease the rates of infection include use of antiseptic skin preparation, antimicrobial prophylaxis (AMP), thermoregulation, and following a sterile technique.[1] Skin preparation with chlorhexidine-alcohol is preferred to povidone-iodine for preventing SSIs.[14] The goals of AMP are to achieve inhibitory concentrations at the incision site and to maintain adequate levels of antimicrobial agents for the duration of surgery. Antimicrobial agents should be administered intravenously no more than 1 hour before making the skin incision.[2,11,12,15,16] If the duration of the procedure exceeds the expected duration of adequate tissue levels or 2 half-lives of the prophylactic antibiotic, an additional dose of the antibiotic should be administered.[1] For cefazolin, the most commonly used prophylactic antibiotic, a repeat dose should be given if the duration of surgery exceeds 3 hours.[2] An additional dose of the antibiotic should be administered in case the estimated blood loss is more than 1500 mL.[3] For patients weighing more than 80 kg, the dose of cefazolin should be doubled to 2 g. With current AMP practices, the rate of postoperative infections has decreased by approximately 50%.[15,17,18]

AMP is recommended for all types of hysterectomies and induced abortion.[19–21] For hysterectomy, cefazolin is the most commonly used AMP agent. Preoperative administration of doxycycline is recommended for women who are undergoing surgically induced abortion.[20,22,23] Gynecologic surgeries for which AMP is not routinely recommended include diagnostic or operative hysteroscopy, endometrial ablation,[24] abdominal myomectomy, and laparoscopy without hysterectomy.[25]

AMP

Cephalosporins are the most widely used AMP agents. This class of antibiotics is effective against gram-positive and gram-negative microorganisms. Secondary to coverage of the more common microorganisms associated with gynecologic SSIs, cefazolin is the first choice for most clean-contaminated procedures.[11,12,15] Cephalosporins are not active against *Enterococci* spp.

If immediate hypersensitivity reaction to penicillin or cephalosporins is reported in patients, use of alternative broad-spectrum AMP agents is recommended. The American College of Obstetrics and Gynecology recommends a combination of non–β-lactam antibiotics. These combinations include clindamycin and gentamicin, clindamycin and ciprofloxacin, clindamycin and aztreonam, metronidazole and gentamicin, or metronidazole and ciprofloxacin.[26] In patients with known history of MRSA infection or colonization, vancomycin, in addition to the preferred agent, is the AMP agent of choice. Vancomycin requires an infusion time of 1 hour (**Table 1**).[1,16]

Appropriate use of a single dose of AMP agent minimizes the potential for emerging microbial resistance.[5,16] Another rare concern after AMP is the development of gastrointestinal overgrowth of *Clostridium difficile*, which can lead to diarrhea, pseudomembranous enterocolitis, and potentially fatal toxic megacolon.[2,10,27] Routine administration of prophylactic antibiotics for the purpose of preventing endocarditis is no longer recommended for gynecologic surgeries.[28]

TYPES AND LOCATIONS OF SSIs

Incisional cellulitis presents with erythema, warmth from the incision, swelling, and/or localized pain. It is not associated with a fluid collection and does not require drainage. The most common organisms associated include *S aureus*, coagulase-negative staphylococci, and streptococci. Incisional cellulitis without abscess frequently responds to oral antimicrobial therapy alone.[15] Vaginal cuff cellulitis after hysterectomy is characterized by induration, erythema, and edema of the cuff.[7,17] In the absence of a cuff abscess, cuff cellulitis can also be treated with oral therapy (**Table 2**).

SSIs are categorized as superficial incisional, deep incisional, and involving organ/space and have been defined by the CDC NNIS system.[29] A superficial incisional SSI or wound infection occurs within 30 days of surgery and involves only the skin or subcutaneous tissue. At least one of the following findings must be present: purulent drainage; culture isolation of an organism from the incision; or symptoms of pain, tenderness, erythema, edema, or warmth from the incision. Deep incisional SSI occurs within 30 days of the surgery and involves the deep soft tissues, such as fascia and

Table 1			
Recommended AMP for gynecologic surgery			
Procedure	**Preferred Antibiotic**	**Dose**	**Alternative Antibiotic and Intravenous Dose**
Hysterectomy	Cefazolin	1–2 g	Cefotetan, 1 g
			Clindamycin, 600 mg; or metronidazole, 500 mg; with gentamicin, 1.5 mg/kg
			Clindamycin, 600 mg; or metronidazole, 500 mg; with ciprofloxacin, 400 mg
			Clindamycin, 600 mg; or metronidazole, 500 mg; with aztreonam, 1 g
Induced Abortion	Doxycycline	100 mg	Metronidazole, 500 mg

Data from Refs.[7,10,26]

Table 2
Recommended oral antibiotic therapies for outpatient management of wound cellulitis

Skin and Soft Tissue Infections	Suggested Antimicrobial Therapies
Skin Cellulitis, Low Suspicion of MRSA	Cephalexin, 500 mg po qid Dicloxacillin, 500 mg po qid Ciprofloxacin, 500 mg po bid
Skin Cellulitis, Concern for MRSA	Trimethoprim-sulfamethoxazole, DS po bid Doxycycline, 100 mg po bid Clindamycin, 300 mg po tid
Vaginal Cuff Cellulitis	Amoxicillin/clavulanate, 875/125 mg po bid Ciprofloxacin, 500 mg po bid; with metronidazole, 500 mg po bid Trimethoprim-sulfamethoxazole, DS po bid with metronidazole, 500 mg po bid

Abbreviation: DS, double strength.
Data from Stevens DL, Bisno AL, Chambers HF, et al. Practice guidelines for the diagnosis and management of skin and soft-tissue infections. Clin Infect Dis 2005;41(10):1373–406.

muscle layers. One of the following findings is required for diagnosis: purulent drainage; a spontaneous dehiscence of a deep incision; the incision is opened due to signs of fever (temperature, >38°C), localized pain, or tenderness; or an abscess or other evidence of deep infection is found. An organ/space SSI (includes surgical site cellulitis, eg, vaginal cuff cellulitis and pelvic abscess, including vaginal cuff abscess or tubo-ovarian abscess [TOA]) occurs within 30 days of surgery, and the infection involves any part of the anatomy other than the incision that was manipulated during surgery. At least one of the following is required: purulent drainage from a drain placed within the organ/space, culture isolation of an organism from the organ/space, an abscess or other infections located within the organ/space, or diagnosis is made by the surgeon.[1]

The most serious form of SSI is necrotizing fasciitis. This infection usually presents with pain disproportionate to physical examination, a thin dishwater drainage, and possible skin bullae. Necrotizing fasciitis is often caused by a polymicrobial infection and can lead to the rapid destruction and necrosis of the surrounding tissue, ultimately resulting in sepsis and end-organ damage. This life-threatening infection requires immediate wide local debridement of affected tissue after the initiation of broad-spectrum parenteral antibiotics.[15]

DIAGNOSIS

The most common complication after hysterectomy is pelvic infection.[17] Patients with SSIs often present with pain and tenderness at the operative site and fever. Postoperative fever after gynecologic surgery is not uncommon in the first 24 hours. Patients with temperature greater than 38.4°C (101°F) in the first 24 hours or greater than 38°C (100.4°F) on 2 occasions at least 4 hours apart excluding the first 24 postoperative hours should be evaluated for infection. On examination, skin erythema, subcutaneous induration, and/or spontaneous drainage of serous or purulent fluid are noted. Pelvic examination may reveal extraordinary vaginal cuff, paravaginal, or pelvic organ tenderness. In case of vaginal cuff abscess, a mass may be palpated at the apex of the vagina. Laboratory tests to evaluate wound infection should include a complete blood count. Leukocytosis of more than 13,000 cells/mm^3 with or without bandemia and increased percentage of polymorphonuclear neutrophils may support the diagnosis of infection. Gram stain and culture from the incision or abscess drainage can be invaluable in directing antimicrobial therapy.[15] Bacteremia is rare[7,30]; therefore, blood cultures need not be routinely obtained in the presence of a postoperative febrile morbidity workup unless the patient appears septic.[30]

IMAGING

When organ/space SSIs are suspected, radiologic evaluation with computed tomography (CT) scan, magnetic resonance imaging (MRI), or ultrasonography can be used to localize the area of infection.[15] Ultrasonography is the least-expensive method for identifying a TOA and is well tolerated by patients. The sensitivity and specificity of ultrasonography in the identification of postoperative intra-abdominal abscess is 81% and 91%, respectively. The classic appearance of a TOA on ultrasonography is a homogenous, cystic, thin-walled contiguous mass.[31] CT findings characteristic of a TOA include multiloculated, thick, uniform, enhancing abscess wall with fluid densities.[32] The appearance of TOA on MRI is similar to CT, demonstrating thick-walled masses with multiple internal septa, shading, and gas collection. The sensitivity and specificity of MRI for the diagnosis of TOA are 95% and 89%, respectively.[33,34] The appearance of a postoperative pelvic abscess is similar to that of a TOA, whether or not the adnexa are involved.

TREATMENT

Not all patients with superficial incisional infections require hospitalization. Patients with a mild wound cellulitis without evidence of a wound abscess or necrotizing fasciitis can be treated as outpatients with oral therapy. Most deep incisional SSIs will require hospitalization and parenteral therapy. The physician should use clinical judgment to determine if a patient can be managed as an outpatient when initiating therapy for the wound infection. Admission should be considered in case of fever with temperature greater than 101F, evidence of peritonitis, intra-abdominal or pelvic abscess, inability to tolerate oral antibiotics, hypotension, or other physical or laboratory indicators of sepsis. In patients requiring hospital admission, parenteral therapy should be initiated (**Table 3**).

Antimicrobial therapy should be directed at the common microbial pathogens associated with postoperative gynecologic infection. For incisional cellulitis, antibiotic therapy should cover gram-positive cocci. In case of localized wound infection, incision and drainage is indicated. In regions where MRSA is prevalent or a concern, antibiotic selection should reflect this. Vaginal cuff cellulitis therapy should be more broad spectrum, covering gram-positive cocci, anaerobes, and gram-negative enterics (see **Table 2** and **Table 3**).

Patients requiring admission should receive parenteral antibiotics. In case of deep incisional or organ/space infections, broad-spectrum antibiotic therapy should be initiated (see **Table 3**). Parenteral antibiotics should be continued until the patient is afebrile and clinically well for at least 24 to 48 hours. If patients do not demonstrate systemic improvement and if there is no resolution of fever within 48 hours, it is recommended to consider repeating the imaging to determine if an abscess is present and/or changing antimicrobials. Drug fever should be considered in well-appearing, stable patients with persistent fever with or without eosinophilia.[15] Septic pelvic thrombophlebitis occurs rarely. It is a diagnosis of exclusion and should be considered in postoperative febrile patients who are not responding to broad-spectrum

Table 3
Recommended parenteral antibiotic therapies for wound and pelvic infections

Skin and Soft Tissue Infections	Suggested Antimicrobial Therapies
Superficial SSI (Wound Infection)	Cefazolin, 1–2 g IV q 6h Ceftriaxone, 1–2 g IV q 24h Cefoxitin, 2 g IV q 6h Ampicillin/sulbactam, 3 g IV q 6h Piperacillin/tazobactam, 3.375 g IV q 6h

Deep/Organ SSI (Cuff Cellulitis, Vaginal Cuff Abscess, TOA, and/or Pelvic Abscess)	Clindamycin, 900 mg IV q 8h; and
	  gentamicin, 5 mg/kg IV q 24h or
	  1.5–2 mg/kg IV q 8h
	Ceftriaxone, 2 g IV q 24h; and clindamycin,
	  900 mg IV q 8h
	Ampicillin, 2 g IV q 4h; and gentamicin,
	  5 mg/kg IV q 24h or 1.5–2 mg/kg IV q 8h;
	  and metronidazole, 500 mg IV q 8h
	  or clindamycin, 900 mg IV q 8h
	Ciprofloxacin, 400 mg IV q 12h; and
	  metronidazole, 500 mg IV q 8h
	Piperacillin/tazobactam, 3.375 g IV q 6h
	Doripenem, 500 mg IV q 8h
	In cases of MRSA infection, add vancomycin,
	  20 mg/kg IV q 12h

Abbreviation: IV, intravenous.
Data from Larsen JW, Hager WD, Livengood CH, et al. Guidelines for the diagnosis, treatment and prevention of postoperative infections. Infect Dis Obstet Gynecol 2003;11(1):65–70.

antibiotics, in the absence of an abscess or hematoma. Treatment may include continuation of antibiotics and the addition of the intravenous heparin.[7]

SURGICAL MANAGEMENT

Superficial incisional abscesses should be opened wide and allowed to drain. The fascia should be probed to rule out dehiscence. Necrotic tissue within the incision should be debrided. After debridement, wound healing may be facilitated with packing, wound vacuum, or secondary closure after adequate regranulation. In the presence of deep incisional and organ/space infections, debridement and drainage are occasionally required. Vaginal cuff abscesses can be accessed by opening the vaginal cuff and probing bluntly to break apart adhesions and allow pus and hematomas to drain. Pelvic and abdominal abscesses may be accessed either surgically or radiologically with CT assistance or ultrasound-guided needle or catheter.[15]

REFERENCES

1. Mangram AJ, Horan TC, Pearson ML, et al. Guideline for prevention of surgical site infection, 1999. Hospital infection control practices advisory committee. Infect Control Hosp Epidemiol 1999;20(4):250–78 [quiz: 79–80].
2. Hemsell DL. Prophylactic antibiotics in gynecologic and obstetric surgery. Rev Infect Dis 1991;13(Suppl 10):S821–41.
3. DiLuigi AJ, Peipert JF, Weitzen S, et al. Prophylactic antibiotic administration prior to hysterectomy: a quality improvement initiative. J Reprod Med 2004;49(12): 949–54.

4. Wenzel RP. Minimizing surgical-site infections. N Engl J Med 2010;362(1):75–7.
5. Duff P, Park RC. Antibiotic prophylaxis in vaginal hysterectomy: a review. Obstet Gynecol 1980;55(Suppl 5):193S–202.
6. Soper DE. Bacterial vaginosis and postoperative infections. Am J Obstet Gynecol 1993;169(2 Pt 2):467–9.
7. Hager WD. Postoperative infections: prevention and management. 9th edition. Philadelphia: Lippincott Williams and Wilkins; 2003.
8. Larsson PG, Carlsson B. Does pre- and postoperative metronidazole treatment lower vaginal cuff infection rate after abdominal hysterectomy among women with bacterial vaginosis? Infect Dis Obstet Gynecol 2002;10(3):133–40.
9. Soper DE, Bump RC, Hurt WG. Bacterial vaginosis and trichomoniasis vaginitis are risk factors for cuff cellulitis after abdominal hysterectomy. Am J Obstet Gynecol 1990;163(3):1016–21 [discussion: 21–3].
10. Kernodle DS, Kaiser A. Surgical and trauma-related infections. 5th edition. Philadephia: Churchill Livingstone; 2000.
11. Tanos V, Rojansky N. Prophylactic antibiotics in abdominal hysterectomy. J Am Coll Surg 1994;179(5):593–600.
12. Peipert JF, Weitzen S, Cruickshank C, et al. Risk factors for febrile morbidity after hysterectomy. Obstet Gynecol 2004;103(1):86–91.
13. Bode LG, Kluytmans JA, Wertheim HF, et al. Preventing surgical-site infections in nasal carriers of Staphylococcus aureus. N Engl J Med 2010;362(1):9–17.
14. Darouiche RO, Wall Jr. MJ, Itani KM, et al. Chlorhexidine-alcohol versus povidone-iodine for surgical-site antisepsis. N Engl J Med 2010;362(1):18–26.
15. Larsen JW, Hager WD, Livengood CH, et al. Guidelines for the diagnosis, treatment and prevention of postoperative infections. Infect Dis Obstet Gynecol 2003;11(1):65–70.
16. Bratzler DW, Houck PM. Antimicrobial prophylaxis for surgery: an advisory statement from the national surgical infection prevention project. Clin Infect Dis 2004;38(12):1706–15.
17. Hemsell DL. Gynecologic postoperative infections. New York: Raven Press; 1994.
18. Mittendorf R, Aronson MP, Berry RE, et al. Avoiding serious infections associated with abdominal hysterectomy: a meta-analysis of antibiotic prophylaxis. Am J Obstet Gynecol 1993;169(5):1119–24.
19. McCausland VM, Fields GA, McCausland AM, et al. Tuboovarian abscesses after operative hysteroscopy. J Reprod Med 1993;38(3):198–200.
20. Moller BR, Allen J, Toft B, et al. Pelvic inflammatory disease after hysterosalpingography associated with Chlamydia trachomatis and Mycoplasma hominis. Br J Obstet Gynaecol 1984;91(12):1181–7.
21. Goldstein S. Sonohysterography. New York: Churchill Livingstone; 1995.
22. Sawaya GF, Grady D, Kerlikowske K, et al. Antibiotics at the time of induced abortion: the case for universal prophylaxis based on a meta-analysis. Obstet Gynecol 1996;87(5 Pt 2):884–90.
23. Pittaway DE, Winfield AC, Maxson W, et al. Prevention of acute pelvic inflammatory disease after hysterosalpingography: efficacy of doxycycline prophylaxis. Am J Obstet Gynecol 1983;147(6):623–6.
24. Bhattacharya S, Parkin DE, Reid TM, et al. A prospective randomised study of the effects of prophylactic antibiotics on the incidence of bacteraemia following hysteroscopic surgery. Eur J Obstet Gynecol Reprod Biol 1995;63(1):37–40.
25. Kocak I, Ustun C, Emre B, et al. Antibiotics prophylaxis in laparoscopy. Ceska Gynekol 2005;70(4):269–72.

26. ACOG Committee on Practice Bulletins–Gynecology. ACOG practice bulletin no. 104: antibiotic prophylaxis for gynecologic procedures. Obstet Gynecol 2009; 113(5):1180–9.

27. Garey KW, Jiang ZD, Yadav Y, et al. Peripartum *Clostridium difficile* infection: case series and review of the literature. Am J Obstet Gynecol 2008;199(4):332–7.

28. Wilson W, Taubert KA, Gewitz M, et al. Prevention of infective endocarditis: guidelines from the American Heart Association: a guideline from the American Heart Association Rheumatic fever, Endocarditis, and Kawasaki Disease Committee, Council on Cardiovascular Disease in the Young, and the Council on Clinical Cardiology, Council on Cardiovascular Surgery and Anesthesia, and the Quality of Care and Outcomes Research Interdisciplinary Working Group. Circulation 2007;116(15):1736–54.

29. Horan TC, Gaynes RP, Martone WJ, et al. CDC definitions of nosocomial surgical site infections: a modification of CDC definitions of surgical wound infections. Infect Control Hosp Epidemiol 1992;13(10):606–8.

30. de la Torre SH, Mandel L, Goff BA. Evaluation of postoperative fever: usefulness and cost-effectiveness of routine workup. Am J Obstet Gynecol 2003;188(6): 1642–7.

31. Moir C, Robins RE. Role of ultrasonography, Gallium scanning, and computed tomography in the diagnosis of intraabdominal abscess. Am J Surg 1982; 143(5):582–5.

32. Hiller N, Sella T, Lev-Sagi A, et al. Computed tomographic features of tuboovarian abscess. J Reprod Med 2005;50(3):203–8.

33. Tukeva TA, Aronen HJ, Karjalainen PT, et al. MR imaging in pelvic inflammatory disease: comparison with laparoscopy and US. Radiology 1999;210(1):209–16.

34. Ha HK, Lim GY, Cha ES, et al. MR imaging of tubo-ovarian abscess. Acta Radiol 1995;36(5):510–4.

Avoiding Major Vessel Injury During Laparoscopic Instrument Insertion

Stephanie D. Pickett, MD[a], Katherine J. Rodewald, MD[a],
Megan R. Billow, DO[a], Nichole M. Giannios, DO[a],
William W. Hurd, MD, MSc[b,c],*

KEYWORDS

- Laparoscopy • Intraoperative complications
- Blood vessel injuries

Laparoscopy is one of the most common surgical approaches performed in the United States today. This surgical approach has gained popularity compared with traditional laparotomy due to increased safety, better outcomes, and shorter recovery periods. Each year gynecologists and general surgeons perform an estimated 2 million laparoscopic procedures, including cholecystectomies, tubal ligations, appendectomies, hysterectomies, urogynecologic repairs, and cancer staging, to name a few.[1] Advances in laparoscopic technology and the development of robotic surgery are likely to further increase the number of cases performed laparoscopically. Fortunately, major complications related to laparoscopy are uncommon, occurring in less than 2% of procedures.[2]

One of the most serious laparoscopic complications is injury to major vessels, which reportedly occurs in approximately 0.04% of cases.[3] Vessel injury occurs most commonly while gaining intra-abdominal access during insertion of the Veress needle and port trocars through the abdominal wall.[2,4] Although vessel injury occurrence is low, mortality is high. Injury to one or more major vessels can quickly result in fatal exsanguinations, with a majority of these deaths occurring within the first 24 hours

The authors have nothing to disclose.

[a] Department of Obstetrics and Gynecology, University Hospitals Case Medical Center, 11100 Euclid Avenue MAC 5034, Cleveland, OH 44106, USA

[b] Division of Reproductive Endocrinology and Infertility, Department of Obstetrics and Gynecology, University Hospitals Case Medical Center, 11100 Euclid Avenue MAC 5034, Cleveland, OH 44106, USA

[c] Department of Reproductive Biology, Case Western Reserve University School of Medicine, 11100 Euclid Avenue MAC 5034, Cleveland, OH 44106, USA

* Corresponding author.

E-mail address: William.Hurd@uhhospitals.org

Obstet Gynecol Clin N Am 37 (2010) 387–397

doi:10.1016/j.ogc.2010.05.002

obgyn.theclinics.com

of surgery.[1] Despite decades of research and development in an effort to create safer instruments, the incidence of these injuries has not decreased.[2,4]

The purpose of this article is to review recommended methods for avoiding major vessel injury while gaining laparoscopic access. A first step is to review the anatomic relationships of abdominal wall landmarks to the major retroperitoneal vessels. Because Veress needles are commonly used to insufflate the abdomen before trocar placement, methods for their successful placement are reviewed. Various methods and locations for primary trocar placement are compared. Finally, methods to avoid vessel injury during placement of secondary ports are described.

MAJOR VESSELS AT RISK DURING LAPAROSCOPY
Major Vessels of the Lower Abdomen and Pelvis

The major arteries that lie in the retroperitoneal space of the lower abdomen and pelvis include the descending aorta, the common iliac arteries, and the external and internal iliac arteries (**Fig. 1**).[5] At the bifurcation, the common iliac arteries diverge bilaterally. Near the pelvic brim, the internal iliac artery branches off dorsally, and the external iliac artery continues caudally to enter the inguinal canal. The inferior epigastic vessels arise from the external iliac arteries and ascend upward through the tranversalis fascia and then between the rectus abdominis and the posterior lamellar sheath.

Analogous venous vessels include the inferior vena cava, common iliac veins, and their internal and external branches. The major veins lie dorsal to these arteries in the lower abdomen and pelvis. Analogous to the arteries, the vena cava bifurcates

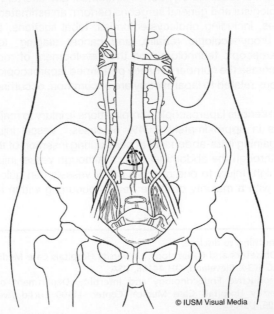

© IUSM Visual Media

Fig. 1. Location of the major vessels in relation to the umbilicus and pelvic bones. The average location of the umbilicus below the aortic bifurcation is indicated by a dashed circle. The major tributaries of the vena cava (ie, the common, internal, and external iliac veins) lie dorsal and medial to the major branches of the aorta (ie, the common, internal, and external iliac arteries). (*From* Sandadi S, Johannigman JA, Wong V, et al. Recognition and management of major vessel injury during laparoscopy. J Minim Invasive Gynecol, 2010, in press; with permission.)

into the common iliac veins. The internal and external iliac veins lie dorsal and medial to the corresponding arteries.

Common Major Vessel Injuries

Injuries during laparoscopic entry have been reported to every major vessel in the pelvis. The relative frequency at which major retroperitoneal vessels are injured during laparoscopy is difficult to determine for several reasons. The first reason is that major vessel injuries are uncommon. In addition, the number of major vessel injuries is higher than the reported number because many major vessel injuries are never reported. It is also likely that fatal major vessel injuries are more likely to be reported.

Despite these limitations, review of 75 published injuries in three small series can give some idea of the vessels at greatest risk of injury during laparoscopy.[1,6,7] A notable aspect of these data was that arterial injuries made up 75% (56/75) of the total: 25% involved the aorta and 21% the right common iliac artery. The remaining 29% of these arterial injuries were distributed between the left common iliac artery and the left or right external or internal iliac arteries. The vena cava was injured in 11% (8/75). All other venous injuries were accompanied by injury of the corresponding overlying artery. Although the side of iliac vessel injury was only specified in 30 cases, 73% (22/30) of these injuries occurred on the right.

The large number of aorta and vena cava injuries was surprising, because these vessels lie at or above the umbilicus in most women.[8] Injuries to these vessels are likely to result from inserting periumbilical instruments at angles greater than 45° from the plane of the spine. The preponderance of right iliac vessel injuries might reflect a tendency of surgeons standing on the left side of patients and inserting instruments with the right hand to place instruments in a direction deviated slightly to the right of midline.

AVOIDING MAJOR VESSEL INJURY DURING LAPAROSCOPIC ENTRY

Insertion of the Veress needle and primary trocar for initial entry remains the most hazardous part of laparoscopy, accounting for 40% of all laparoscopic complications and the majority of the fatalities.[1] Despite decades of research and development to find safer methods for initial laparoscopic entry, major vessel injuries have been reported using virtually all types of trocar insertion methods.[9]

The first modern laparoscopic entry techniques used to gain laparoscopic access used a periumbilical insertion site and were categorized as closed or open. The traditional closed technique involves blind placement of a Veress needle and sharp primary trocar, whereas the open technique is performed by placing a blunt trocar through a minilaparotomy incision. Other techniques that have been developed include direct trocar insertion (a closed technique where the primary trocar is inserted before peritoneal insufflation), left upper quadrant (LUQ) insertion (where an alternate insertion site is used), and the use of innovative trocar designs. Some of the most commonly reported methods are compared.

Closed Laparoscopy: Veress Needle and Primary Trocar

The majority of retroperitoneal vessel injuries during laparoscopy occur during blind placement of the Veress needle or primary trocar through a periumbilical incision.[4] To minimize this risk, surgeons should have an accurate understanding of the anatomy of the lower abdomen and pelvis.[10]

Traditionally, the primary site of entry into the abdomen is located in the midsagital plane at the lower margin or base of the umbilicus. This location was originally chosen for cosmetic and safety reasons. There are no major blood vessels in the midline of the pelvis because the aorta and vena cava bifurcate near the umbilicus. Thus, placing the Verres needle and primary trocar through the umbilicus directed toward the pelvis was found to be safe.[11] This safety depends, however, on appropriate direction and angle of insertion.

Direction of insertion

The umbilicus is an excellent anatomic landmark to determine the midline. Instruments placed through the umbilicus must be inserted, however, in a direction parallel to the long axis of the patient so that their sharp tips remain in the midline. A deviation of as little as 20 mm from parallel places an instrument tip almost 4 cm from the midline.

To minimize the risk of major vessel injuries when placing instruments through the umbilicus, every effort must be made to keep the direction of insertion in the midline. Unfortunately, the long axis of a patient can be difficult to estimate after the patient has been covered in drapes. The propensity of right-sided major vessel injuries (described previously) is probably related to this difficulty.

Angle of insertion

A second variable to consider when inserting laparoscopic instruments through the umbilicus is the angle of insertion. Based on the location of the major vessels and their bifurcations, the standard approach in the early years of laparoscopy was to place the Veress needle and primary trocar through the umbilicus 45° from the horizontal plane of a patient's spine.[12] It became apparent, however, that in obese patients, instruments inserted at this angle would often not enter the peritoneal cavity. For this reason, some surgeons recommended inserting instruments at 90° from the horizontal plane in obese patients[13] and other surgeons recommend this angle in all patients.[9]

An anatomic study subsequently illustrated that the anatomy of the abdominal wall changed greatly with weight and thus the angle of insertion should be modified accordingly (**Fig. 2**).[10] For practical purposes, women can be divided into nonobese (includes normal weight and overweight) and obese categories. Nonobese women have a body mass index less than or equal to 30 kg/m², whereas obese women have a body mass index greater than 30 kg/m², which corresponds to a weight greater

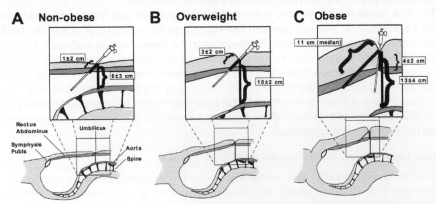

Fig. 2. Changes in the anatomy of the anterior abdominal wall based on weight. (*From* Hurd WW, Bude RO, DeLancey JO, et al. Abdominal wall characterization with magnetic resonance imaging and computed tomography. The effect of obesity on the laparoscopic approach. J Reprod Med 1991;36:473–6; with permission.)

than 91 kg (>200 lb). The ideal angles of insertion based on weight are based on these data.

In nonobese women, it is recommended that instruments be inserted through the umbilicus at 45° from the horizontal plane of a patient's spine. At this angle, the abdominal wall thickness in nonobese women ranges from an average of 2 to 3 cm; thus, successful intraperitoneal placement of instruments is highly likely (see **Fig. 2**A, B). This angle is also likely to minimize the risk of major vessel injury, because the distance from the skin to these vessels at 90° averages only 6 to 10 cm and can be as close as 2 cm in slender patients. In addition, the aortic bifurcation is often at or caudal to the level of the umbilicus in nonobese patients.[8]

In obese women, it is recommended that instruments be inserted through the umbilicus closer to 90° from the horizontal plane of a patient's spine. At 45°, the abdominal wall thickness in obese women is often greater than 11 cm, making successful intraperitoneal placement unlikely (see **Fig. 2**C). Fortunately, the distance from the skin to these vessels at 90° averages greater than 13 cm, and the aortic bifurcation is almost always cephalad to the level of the umbilicus in obese patients.[8]

To place instruments through the umbilicus at the proper angle, it is important to be aware of a patient's position in relation to horizontal.[6] Most laparoscopic surgery is performed in the Trendelenburg position (feet higher than the head) to keep bowel away from the operative field in the pelvis. If a patient is placed in Trendelenburg position with the feet elevated 30° relative to the head before instrument insertion, instruments inserted at 45° from horizontal are placed at 75° from the horizontal plane of the patient's spine. This is likely to increase the risk of major vessel injury, particularly in slender patients.[6] For greatest safety, surgeons should make sure they are aware of a patient's position in relation to horizontal before laparoscopic instrument placement.

High-pressure entry

Another technique used in conjunction with closed laparoscopy in an effort to decrease the risk of major vessel injury is high-pressure entry. Rather than inserting the primary umbilical trocar after obtaining intra-abdominal pressure of 18 to 20 mm Hg, many surgeons increase the pressure to 25 to 30 mm Hg. The rationale is to make the anterior abdominal wall stiffer such that the downward pressure exerted by trocar insertion does not decrease the distance of the umbilicus to the retroperitoneal vessels.[14] Although no controlled studies large enough to demonstrate an advantage have been published, large series, including more than 8000 cases, suggest that the risk of major vessel injury using this technique is approximately 1 in 10,000 cases (0.01%) compared with a risk of 4 in 10,000 cases (0.04%) reported using standard pressures.[13,14]

Verify location of Veress needle tip

A Veress needle is used to insufflate the peritoneal cavity before trocar insertion by the majority of gynecologists.[15] One disadvantage of using a Veress needle is that it dramatically increases the risk of intravascular insufflation and venous gas embolism, a rare complication of laparoscopic entry, reported to occur in approximately 1 in 100,00 cases.[16]

To prevent intravascular insufflation when using a Veress needle, it is recommended that efforts be made to verify that the tip of the needle is located in the peritoneal cavity before insufflation.[2] The following maneuvers have been proposed minimize the risk of intravascular insufflation.

- The Veress needle value should be open when the needle is inserted. Spontaneous egress of fresh blood through the needle indicates that the tips had entered an artery.
- The double-click test. A surgeon should feel or hear two clicks as a Veress needle is placed through the abdominal wall. The retracted blunt needle tip will suddenly extend after it passes through the anterior rectus abdominus fascia and again when it enters the peritoneal cavity.[2]
- The waggle test. The hub of the Veress needle should move freely about a fulcrum point located within the anterior abdominal wall. Lack of free movement suggests that the needle tip has entered an intraperitoneal or retroperitoneal structure and the needle should be partially withdrawn. Opponents of this maneuver point out that, if done forcefully, it is likely to enlarge an injury to a fixed vessel or viscus.[17] It is also likely, however, to alert surgeons to the possibility of retroperitoneal placement before insufflation.
- The aspiration test. The Veress needle should be aspirated with a 5-mL syringe after placement. Aspiration of fresh blood fresh blood through the needle suggests that the tips had entered a vein.[2]
- The drop test. A drop of saline is placed in the opened hub of the Veress needle, and the abdominal wall is lifted. If the drop is drawn into the hub, it is likely that the needle tip is in the abdominal cavity.[18] If not, it might suggest that the location of the needle tip is preperitoneal (most likely), retroperitoneal, or within a viscus.

It is recommended that one or more of these methods be used when placing a Veress needle into the abdomen.[18] None of these methods, however, absolutely assures intraperitoneal placement of the needle tip, and it is unlikely that any of them can completely prevent intravascular insufflation. Once insufflation is begun, the strongest predictor of intraperitoneal placement seems to be an initial filling pressure of less than 10 mm Hg.[19]

Open Laparoscopy

Open laparoscopy is the most widely used alternative technique for placement of the primary laparoscopic port. The Hasson technique is fundamentally a minilaparotomy incision followed by placement of the primary port directly into the peritoneal cavity.[20] This avoids the blind placement of the Veress needle and sharp trocar. Instead, the periumbilical fascia is incised with a scalpel or scissors, the peritoneum entered bluntly, and the primary port is placed into the peritoneal cavity using a blunt trocar.

Open laparoscopy has been demonstrated to decrease, but not completely prevent, the risk of major vessel injury.[21] Although early studies suggested that the open technique completely avoided major vessel injuries, subsequent studies found that the open technique decreased the rate of vascular injury to 0.01% compared with a rate of 0.04% associated with closed techniques using a Veress needle.[3] To date, no case of intravascular insufflation has been reported using an open technique. Most gynecologists continue to use a closed technique, however, because major vessel injury remains rare and large studies have not demonstrated a decreased risk of bowel injuries using the open technique.[22]

Other Laparoscopic Entry Methods

Multiple insertion methods and instruments have been developed in the past 20 years in an effort to decrease the risk of trocar complications, most notably injuries to bowel or major blood vessels. Each method seems to have theoretic advantages compared with the traditional closed and open techniques. None, however, seems to have completely eliminated the risk of major vessel injury.

Direct trocar insertion

Direct trocar insertion is a laparoscopic entry technique wherein the primary trocar is placed without prior insufflation.[23] The advantages of direct trocar insertion are that this technique is slightly faster than standard closed laparoscopy and avoids the risks of Veress needle placement. For this technique, the primary trocar is inserted though the umbilicus, with or without elevation of the anterior abdominal wall manually or with towel clips.[24]

Although no controlled studies of direct trocar insertion have been published that are large enough to demonstrate the relative risk of major vessel injury, it seems that this technique might actually increase this risk. Larger series, including more than 10,000 cases, suggest a risk of major vessel injuries in the range of 0.06% to 0.09% of cases compared with a risk of 0.04% of cases reported using a standard closed technique.[3,25,26] This observation is not surprising. If high pressure abdominal insufflation resists downward pressure exerted by trocar insertion and helps maintain the distance of the umbilicus to the retroperitoneal vessels, it makes sense that no abdominal insufflation might increase the risk of the trocar tip coming into contact with retroperitoneal structures.[14] This apparent increased risk of major vessel injury might be one reason why direct trocar insertion is one of the least frequently used techniques by gynecologists.[3]

Left upper quadrant insertion

Insertion of the Veress needle and primary trocar through a site in the LUQ is recommended by some surgeons to decrease the risk of complications associated with bowel adhesions in women with prior abdominal surgeries.[27,28] The LUQ insertion site (Palmer point) is located 3 cm below the middle of the left costal margin, and instruments are routine inserted perpendicular to patients' skin.[29]

The risk of major vessel injury using the LUQ technique remains uncertain. No major vessel injuries have been reported to date, at least in part because to date fewer than 2000 cases using this technique have been published. Anatomic studies indicate that the abdominal wall is uniformly thin in this location and the distance from the skin to the retroperitoneal structures is greater than 11 cm in most patients.[30] Because this distance can be less than 7 cm in many slender patients, however, it is recommended that instruments placed through the Palmer point in slender patients be directed 45° caudally in relation to a patient's spine.[30]

Alternative primary trocars

Multiple innovative primary trocars have been developed over the past 20 years in an effort to decrease entry complications. Most notable among these are shielded disposable trocars, optical trocars, and radially expanding trocars.[31–33] Although studies of these methods have not demonstrated a dramatic increase in complications compared with the traditional closed technique, major blood vessel injuries seem to remain a risk of primary trocar insertion.[2,34] Published controlled studies have uniformly been underpowered to determine the relative risk of major vessel injures associated with these techniques because of the rarity of these events. Thus, there is currently no evidence of benefit of one technique or instrument over another in terms of preventing major vascular injury.[2,35]

AVOIDING VESSEL INJURY DURING SECONDARY PORT TROCAR PLACEMENT
Initial Insertion of Secondary Ports

Major vessel injuries can also occur during placement of secondary ports, in particular those placed lateral to the midline.[36] Secondary trocars are usually placed 5 cm superior to the midpubic symphysis and 8 cm lateral to the midline in an effort to avoid injury to vessels in the anterior abdominal wall.[37] Unfortunately, this location is often directly over the external iliac vessels. For this reason, great care must be taken when inserting trocars in this location to avoid major vessel injuries. The following methods are based on anatomic data and clinical experience, but none has proved to decrease the risk of major vessel injury.

It is well appreciated that it is important to laparoscopically visualize the tip of secondary trocars during placement.[36] This presupposes that trocars are always placed under ideal control, however. In practice, the variation in density of the abdominal wall layers and trocar protective mechanisms can result in sudden loss of resistance accompanied by unexpectedly vigorous and deep trocar insertion. For this reason, measures should be taken to control direction, depth, and speed during secondary trocars insertion.

Direction

The direction of insertion of secondary port trocars is determined by abdominal wall anatomy and the proximity of underlying structures. Secondary trocars are inserted as close a possible to perpendicular to the abdominal wall and underlying peritoneum for two reasons. First, it is often difficult to penetrate the peritoneum obliquely, and second, oblique placement toward the midline can injure abdominal wall vessel, even when the insertion site is well lateral. In this direction, however, the tip of a lateral port trocar is often pointed directly at the external iliac vessels. For this reason, once the trocar tip has penetrated the peritoneum, the direction of insertion should be changed medially away from these vessels.

Depth

The depth of insertion of secondary port trocars should be limited. The goal is to place the trocar sleeve completely through the abdominal wall peritoneum. Excess depth of insertion is one of the common causes of trocar injuries and is often related to uncontrolled thrust of the trocar into the abdomen after an unexpected loss of resistance.[38] To stop a trocar's forward progress as soon as it has penetrated the peritoneum, it is recommended that surgeons consciously balance the force of the agonist muscles, which produce forward thrust, with the antagonist muscles, which stop it.[38] In the event of an unexpected loss of resistance, the subsequent depth of insertion can also be limited either by extensions of the index finger on the inserting hand or by using a two-hand insertion technique where the second hand grasps the sleeve near the skin.

Speed

Speed of insertion is the final parameter that can be controlled during secondary port placement. To minimize the risk of injury, trocars should be inserted slowly rather than quickly even when there is adequate distance between the compressed abdominal wall and the nearest major vessel.[38] This is particularly important when the distance between the emerging trocar tip and major vessels (or bowel) is limited, so that the retracting blade or extending shield found in many modern trocars can deploy. When trocars without such devices are used, controlled speed allows redirection of the emerging trocar tip away from vital structures (discussed previously).

Reinsertion of Secondary Ports

Major vessel injury can also occur during reinsertion of secondary trocars, particularly when the pneumoperitoneum has been lost.[38] Port reinsertion is required when a port has inadvertently been removed from the peritoneal cavity or when a smaller (5-mm) sleeve must be replaced with a larger (10–12 mm) sleeve for specimen removal. The risk of vessel injury can be almost completely avoided by not using a sharp trocar for reinsertion. There are several possible methods that can be used for this purpose.

A safe method for reinserting a port without using a trocar is to place a laparoscopic instrument (eg, blunt probe or grasper) through the port and into the incision and locating the fascial and peritoneal incisions by gentle probing. Once located, the sleeve can be slid over the instrument, much the same way that a catheter is advanced over a guide wire for placement of a central line into a deep vessel.[11]

Another method for reinsertion of the same-sized port or larger back into an existing port site is by using a blunt trocar.[39] Although specially designed blunt trocars were used for this purpose in the past, several modern trocar designs allow for the blade to be retracted into blunt conical blade guard before reinsertion of the sleeve into the abdomen.

SUMMARY

Laparoscopy offers patients a minimally invasive approach to common gynecologic procedures. It has become an accepted approach for most gynecologic problems. Laparoscopic surgeons should have a thorough understanding of the anatomy of the lower abdomen and pelvis. Although vessel injuries remain rare complications of laparoscopic surgery, surgeons should use techniques that can decrease the risk of these injuries so that patients can enjoy the benefits of minimally invasive surgical techniques.

REFERENCES

1. Fuller J, Ashar BS, Carey-Corrado J. Trocar-associated injuries and fatalities: an analysis of 1399 reports to the FDA. J Minim Invasive Gynecol 2005;12:302–7.
2. Vilos GA, Ternamian A, Dempster J, et al. Laparoscopic entry: a review of techniques, technologies, and complications. J Obstet Gynaecol Can 2007;29:433–65.
3. Molloy D, Kalloo PD, Cooper M, et al. Laparoscopic entry: a literature review and analysis of techniques and complications of primary port entry. Aust N Z J Obstet Gynaecol 2002;42:246–54.
4. Saville LE, Woods MS. Laparoscopy and major retroperitoneal vascular injuries (MRVI). Surg Endosc 1995;9:1096–100.
5. Sandadi S, Johannigman JA, Wong V, et al. Recognition and management of major vessel injury during laparoscopy. J Minim Invasive Gynecol, 2010, in press.
6. Soderstrom RM. Injuries to major blood vessels during endoscopy. J Am Assoc Gynecol Laparosc 1997;4:395–8.
7. Azevedo JL, Azevedo OC, Miyahira SA, et al. Injuries caused by Veress needle insertion for creation of pneumoperitoneum: a systematic literature review. Surg Endosc 2009;23:1428–32.
8. Hurd WW, Bude RO, DeLancey JO, et al. The relationship of the umbilicus to the aortic bifurcation: implications for laparoscopic technique. Obstet Gynecol 1992;80:48–51.

9. Shirk GJ, Johns A, Redwine DB. Complications of laparoscopic surgery: how to avoid them and how to repair them. J Minim Invasive Gynecol 2006;13:352–9.
10. Hurd WW, Bude RO, DeLancey JO, et al. Abdominal wall characterization with magnetic resonance imaging and computed tomography. The effect of obesity on the laparoscopic approach. J Reprod Med 1991;36:473–6.
11. Semm K. Operative manual for endoscopic abdominal surgery. Chicago: Year Book Medical Publishers; 1987. p. 66–9.
12. McBrien MP. The technique of peritoneoscopy. Br J Surg 1971;58:433–6.
13. Loffer FD, Pent D. Laparoscopy in the obese patient. Am J Obstet Gynecol 1976; 125:104–7.
14. Garry R. Towards evidence based laparoscopic entry techniques: clinical problems and dilemmas. Gynaecol Endosc 1999;8:315–26.
15. Jansen FW, Kolkman W, Bakkum EA, et al. Complications of laparoscopy: an inquiry about closed-versus open-entry technique. Am J Obstet Gynecol 2004; 190:634–8.
16. Bonjer HJ, Hazebroek EJ, Kazemier G, et al. Open versus closed establishment of pneumoperitoneum in laparoscopic surgery. Br J Surg 1997;84:599–602.
17. Brosens I, Gordon A. Bowel injuries during gynaecological laparoscopy: a multinational survey. Gynecol Endosc 2001;10:141–5.
18. Teoh B, Sen R, Abbott J. An evaluation of four tests used to ascertain Veres needle placement at closed laparoscopy. J Minim Invasive Gynecol 2005;12:153–8.
19. Vilos AG, Vilos GA, Abu-Rafea B, et al. Effect of body habitus and parity on the initial Veres intraperitoneal (VIP) CO2 insufflation pressure during laparoscopic access in women. J Minim Invasive Gynecol 2006;13:108–13.
20. Hasson HM. A modified instrument and method for laparoscopy. Am J Obstet Gynecol 1971;110:886–7.
21. Hasson HM. Open laparoscopy as a method of access in laparoscopic surgery. Gynecol Endosc 1999;8:353–62.
22. Chapron C, Cravello L, Chopin N, et al. Complications during set-up procedures for laparoscopy in gynecology: open laparoscopy does not reduce the risk of major complications. Acta Obstet Gynecol Scand 2003;82:1125–9.
23. Copeland C, Wing R, Hulka JF. Direct trocar insertion at laparoscopy: an evaluation. Obstet Gynecol 1983;62:655–9.
24. Borgatta L, Gruss L, Barad D, et al. Direct trocar insertion vs. Verres needle use for laparoscopic sterilization. J Reprod Med 1990;35:891–4.
25. Woolcott R. The safety of laparoscopy performed by direct trocar insertion and carbon dioxide insufflation under vision. Aust N Z J Obstet Gynaecol 1997;37: 216–9.
26. Kaali SG, Barad DH. Incidence of bowel injury due to dense adhesions at the sight of direct trocar insertion. J Reprod Med 1992;37:617–8.
27. Agarwala N, Liu CY. Safe entry techniques during laparoscopy: left upper quadrant entry using the ninth intercostal space – a review of 918 procedures. J Minim Invasive Gynecol 2005;12:55–61.
28. Howard FM, El-Minawi AM, DeLoach VE. Direct laparoscopic cannula insertion at the left upper quadrant. J Am Assoc Gynecol Laparosc 1997;4:595–600.
29. Palmer R. Safety in laparoscopy. J Reprod Med 1974;13:1–5.
30. Giannios NM, Rohlck KE, Gulani V, et al. Left upper quadrant laparoscopic instrument placement: effects of insertion angle and body mass index on distance to posterior peritoneum by magnetic resonance imaging. Am J Obstet Gynecol 2009;201:522.

31. Kaali SG. Introduction of the Opti-Trocar. J Am Assoc Gynecol Laparosc 1993;1: 50–3.
32. Mettler L, Schmidt EH, Frank V, et al. Optical trocar systems: laparoscopic entry and its complications (a study of case in Germany). Gynaecol Endosc 1999;8: 383–9.
33. Turner DJ. Making the case for the radially expanding access system. Gynaecol Endosc 1999;8:391–5.
34. Sharp HT, Dodson MK, Draper ML, et al. Complications associated with optical-access laparoscopic trocars. Obstet Gynecol 2002;99:553–5.
35. Ahmad G, Duffy JM, Phillips K, et al. Laparoscopic entry techniques. Cochrane Database Syst Rev 2008;2:CD006583.
36. Schafer M, Lauper M, Krahenbuhl L. Trocar and Veress needle injury during laparoscopy. Surg Endosc 2001;15:275–80.
37. Hurd WW, Bude RO, DeLancey JO, et al. The location of abdominal wall blood vessels in relationship to abdominal landmarks apparent at laparoscopy. Am J Obstet Gynecol 1994;171:642–6.
38. Bhoyrul S, Vierra MA, Nezhat CR, et al. Trocar injuries in laparoscopic surgery. J Am Coll Surg 2001;192:677–83.
39. Davis DR, Schilder JM, Hurd WW. Laparoscopic secondary port conversion using a reusable blunt conical trocar. Obstet Gynecol 2000;96:634–5.

Complications of Hysteroscopic and Uterine Resectoscopic Surgery

Malcolm G. Munro, MD, FRCS(c)[a,b,*]

KEYWORDS

- Hysteroscopy • Electrosurgery • Complications
- Distending media • Risk reduction

Hysteroscopy is the process of visualizing the cervical canal and endometrial cavity with an endoscope. If used only for diagnosis, the procedure is limited to visualization with or without sampling of the endometrium or target lesions in the endometrium and cervical canal. However, hysteroscopy can also be used to guide the performance of a spectrum of intrauterine surgical procedures that include adhesiolysis, metroplasty, myomectomy, polypectomy, sterilization, and endometrial ablation. Such procedures are performed in the context of uterine distension with one of several gas or fluid media, using one or a combination of mechanical and energy-based instruments that are externally manipulated by the surgeon. With appropriate understanding and care of these instruments and attention to meticulous technique, hysteroscopy is extremely safe, with many procedures even suitable for performance in the office procedure room. However, since its introduction to the literature in 1869,[1] it has become apparent that there are several potential complications that, although rare, collectively mandate a systematic approach to the procedure designed to minimize the risk of such adverse events or to facilitate early recognition and prompt management should they occur. As with any procedure, risk management starts with patient counseling that includes a thorough discussion of diagnostic and therapeutic treatment options, and of the spectrum of adverse events that may occur with each, appropriately adjusted to fit the risk profile of the patient.

---

[a] Department of Obstetrics & Gynecology, David Geffen School of Medicine at UCLA, Los Angeles, CA, USA
[b] Department of Obstetrics & Gynecology, Kaiser-Permanente, Los Angeles Medical Center, 4900 Sunset Boulevard, Station 3-B, Los Angeles, CA 90027, USA
* Department of Obstetrics & Gynecology, David Geffen School of Medicine at UCLA, Los Angeles, CA.
E-mail address: mmunro@ucla.edu

Obstet Gynecol Clin N Am 37 (2010) 399–425
doi:10.1016/j.ogc.2010.05.006
0889-8545/10/$ – see front matter © 2010 Elsevier Inc. All rights reserved.

GENERAL CONSIDERATIONS

Hysteroscopic procedures are associated with a low incidence of adverse events, with an incidence reported from the Netherlands as 0.28% of 13,600 procedures,[2] and from Germany as 0.24% of 21,676 cases.[3] In general, it is apparent that complicated procedures are associated with a higher risk, with operations such as metroplasty and myomectomy associated with risks of complications as high as 10%.[4] Even resectoscopic endometrial ablation, a low-risk procedure, is associated with a higher risk of intraoperative complications when a loop electrode is used compared with simple rollerball coagulation.[5]

There is a spectrum of perioperative and late risks of operative hysteroscopy (**Table 1**). Perioperative risks are those related to patient positioning, anesthesia, and access to the endometrial cavity that include cervical trauma and uterine perforation and its sequelae. Such adverse events also include gas (especially air) emboli, intraoperative bleeding, fluid and electrolyte disturbances related to excessive absorption of distention media, and lower genital tract injuries related to diversion of radiofrequency (RF) current during electrosurgery with monopolar instrumentation. Early postoperative complications include infection and postoperative bleeding, whereas late complications may be related to sequelae such as intrauterine adhesions and uterine rupture during a pregnancy. To facilitate discussion of these adverse events, as well as early detection, management, and risk reduction of/for the specific complications, this article discusses the competencies required to perform hysteroscopy.

Table 1
Complications and adverse events of hysteroscopy

Adverse Event Category	
Patient positioning	Neurologic
	Compartment syndrome
Anesthesia	General
	Regional
	Conscious sedation
	Local
Access	Cervical trauma
	Perforation
Distending media	Gas emboli
	Fluid overload
	Electrolyte disturbances
Gas emboli	CO_2
	Air
Perforation	Uterus only
	Adjacent structures (bowel, bladder, vessels)
Bleeding	Cervical
	Endomyometrial
	Pelvic vessels
Electrosurgical	Local (active electrodes)
	Remote (currant diversion)
Infection	Endomyometritis
	Peritonitis
Late complications	Intrauterine adhesions (synechiae)
	Pregnancy-related (uterine rupture, placenta accreta/increta, and so forth)

SPECIFIC COMPLICATIONS

In the operating room, adverse events can be a result of suboptimal or incorrect patient positioning, which is particularly an issue when regional or general anesthesia precludes real-time patient feedback. The first hysteroscopy-specific competency is that of access to the endometrial cavity; when this process goes wrong, the operation cannot even begin. The next component of a hysteroscopic procedure is transitioning the potential space that is the endometrial cavity into a working space that allows the surgeon to work. This transition requires the infusion of any of several distending media, but each has potential issues that can result in undesired outcomes. The use of surgical instruments, including the resectoscope, can result in perforation that, in turn, has the potential to result in damage to surrounding organs, which in this case include bowel, bladder, and nearby blood vessels. Intra- and postoperative bleeding are rarely catastrophic but can frequently compromise the performance of the procedure. Infection is believed to be rare, but there are several issues with RF electrosurgery that are unique to hysteroscopy, and our understanding, although limited, now allows us to better rationalize, and perhaps prevent, adverse outcomes related to this modality. There are several late complications, such as intrauterine adhesions, hematometria, and, in the event of pregnancy, uterine rupture, that may present unique challenges for the patient and the surgeon.

COMPLICATIONS RELATED TO PATIENT POSITIONING
Adverse Events

Nerve trauma, direct trauma, and compartment syndromes are the most commonly encountered complications of patient positioning at laparoscopy. It is likely that most of these adverse events occur in women undergoing prolonged general or regional anesthesia in the lithotomy position.

Background

Complications of the lithotomy or modified lithotomy positions are not unique to hysteroscopy, but must be respected when performing intrauterine endoscopy, particularly if general or regional anesthesia is used. When anesthesia is provided by local technique, patients can report discomfort associated with positioning, thereby reducing, if not eliminating, the risk of positioning-related adverse events.

Acute compartment syndrome
Use of the dorsal lithotomy position has been associated with the development of a postoperative compartment syndrome in the lower legs. Compartment syndrome occurs when the pressure in the muscle of an osteofascial compartment is increased to an extent that compromises local vascular perfusion.[6,7] This period of ischemia is followed by reperfusion, capillary leakage from the ischemic tissue, and a further increase in tissue edema in an ongoing cycle that ultimately results in neuromuscular compromise that can cause rhabdomyolysis and serious sequelae including permanent disability. In the lithotomy position, a variety of intraoperative events may facilitate this process: leg holders, pneumatic compression stockings, and other sources of direct pressure may increase intramuscular pressure. Leg perfusion is inherently reduced in the lithotomy and low lithotomy position, but may be enhanced by extreme hip and knee flexion, and has been shown to be more common in individuals with high body mass index and in cases that are prolonged, usually more than 3 hours in duration.[8]

Neurologic injury

The principal motor nerves arising from the lumbosacral plexus (T12 to S4) are the femoral, the obturator, and the sciatic nerves; the numerous sensory nerves include the iliohypogastric, ilioinguinal, genitofemoral, pudental, femoral, sciatic, and lateral femoral cutaneous nerves. Injury to one or more of these nerves can occur in association with hysteroscopic surgery as it is performed in the lithotomy position. Regardless of the mechanistic problem with patient positioning, the risk of neurologic injury increases with prolonged operative time.[9]

Femoral neuropathy occurs secondary to one or a combination of excessive hip flexion, abduction, and external hip rotation that contribute to extreme angulation (>80°) of the femoral nerve beneath the inguinal ligament and resulting nerve compression.[10] These injuries generally resolve, but it may take months and intensive physical therapy to regain normal baseline function.

The sciatic and peroneal nerves are fixed at the sciatic notch and neck of the fibula respectively, making them susceptible to stretch injury.[11] Two orientations create maximal stretch at these points: flexion of the hip with a straight knee, which essentially positions the entire leg vertically; and extreme external rotation of the thighs at the hip. The sciatic nerve can also be traumatized with excessive hip flexion. The common peroneal nerve is also susceptible to compression injury where it separates from the sciatic nerve and courses laterally over the head of the fibula. If there is excessive pressure over the head of the fibula from, for example, a stirrup, neural injury results in foot drop and lateral lower extremity paresthesia.

Risk Reduction, Recognition, and Management of Adverse Events Related to Patient Positioning

Because neurologic injury and compartment syndrome seem to be related to preoperative patient positioning, and, to some extent, the length of surgery, there is an opportunity to reduce risk with several consistently applied steps and precautions. Ideal lithotomy positioning requires that flexion at the knee and hip be kept moderate, with limited abduction and external rotation. This approach reduces the stretch or compression on the femoral and sciatic nerves. If the legs are positioned in stirrups, it is important to avoid pressure on the femoral head, which can damage the common peroneal nerve. All members of the operative team should avoid leaning on the thigh of the patient, because this can stretch the sciatic nerve.

Surgeons must also recognize the relationship between leg positioning and the development of compartment syndrome, especially in prolonged cases. Steps should be taken to elevate the legs only to the extent necessary, and to position stirrups or boots so that as much of the weight as possible is borne by the foot.

For any of these adverse events, it is important to make a prompt diagnosis to minimize the risk of permanent serious sequelae. With compartment syndrome, decompression techniques can prevent local and systemic long-term sequelae. When neuropathy occurs, it is important to introduce appropriate physical therapy early to reduce the chance of long-term or permanent muscle atrophy, thereby facilitating the ultimate return of normal function.

ANESTHESIA
Adverse Events

As is the case with any surgical procedure performed under regional or general anesthesia, there is a spectrum of generic complications that, in some instances, can be catastrophic. Allergy, systemic injection, and overdose comprise the main adverse events associated with the use of local anesthesia.

Background

Regional and general anesthesia

It is beyond the scope of this article to deal with the spectrum of complications that relate to regional and general anesthesia. However, the anesthesiologist must be aware of issues that may be first appreciated at the head of the operating table. These issues include fluid overload and electrolyte disturbances and the signs of gas embolization, with room air, the products of tissue vaporization, or distending gases such as CO_2. Each of these situations is discussed later in this paper. Issues relating to the use of anxiolytics and systemic analgesics that, alone or in combination, are often called conscious sedation, are also not dealt with. The reader is referred to recent American College of Obstetricians and Gynecologists guidelines on the subject.[12]

Local anesthesia

Local anesthetic agents may be administered by the surgeon to add to the effect of systemic analgesia provided by an anesthesiologist who can provide assistance should adverse events occur. However, in most office settings, such agents are the sole source of anesthesia, and the surgeon is usually the only physician in the room. Consequently, it is incumbent on the surgeon to understand the prevention and management of complications related to these locally active drugs.

Locally active anesthetic agents are generally from the amino amide or amino ester class, the latter being modified versions of *para*-aminobenzoic acid (PABA). These agents alter neuronal depolarization by blocking the sodium channels in the cell membrane, most commonly those of sensory nerves, thereby preventing transmission of the sensation of pain to the higher neurons. In large part, they are metabolized in the liver with a half-life that varies according to the specific agent and several factors discussed later, but typically is in the range of 1.5 to 2 hours.

With judicious use, serious adverse reactions to injectable anesthetics are uncommon, but they have been described in relation to high plasma concentrations that are secondary to one or a combination of: (1) inadvertent intravascular injection, (2) excessive dose, and (3) delayed clearance/metabolism. The potential central nervous system side effects of high plasma levels include mouth tingling, tremor, dizziness, blurred vision, and seizures, and can culminate in respiratory depression and apnea. Cardiovascular side effects are those of direct myocardial depression (bradycardia and potential cardiovascular collapse), an adverse event more commonly described in association with bupivicaine. Allergic reactions are generally immunoglobulin E (IgE)–mediated and are usually associated with the ester class of anesthetics, related to the immunogenicity of PABA. Amino amide anesthetics do not contain PABA, a circumstance that markedly reduces the risk of allergy, making the amides the most commonly used agents.

Topical agents can also be associated with adverse events, including systemic absorption that may be facilitated when the agent is applied to disrupted epithelial surfaces. The local effects may be limited to burning or stinging, whereas systemic effects mirror those associated with injectable agents, although serious and severe manifestations are rare.

Risk Reduction, Recognition, and Management of Local Anesthesia–related Adverse Events

The adverse events associated with the use of injectable local anesthetic agents are virtually eliminated by screening for allergy, and with strict attention to total dosage (in mg/kg) and injection technique, taking care to avoid intravascular injection. The use of solutions with dilute epinephrine reduces the risk and extent of systemic absorption.

Overdosage is prevented by ensuring that intravascular injection is avoided and by not exceeding the maximum recommended doses (lidocaine, 4 mg/kg; mepivacaine, 3 mg/kg). The use of a vasoconstrictor reduces the systemic absorption of the agent, almost doubling the maximum dose that can be used. Complications of intravascular injection or anesthetic overdose include allergy, neurologic effects, and impaired myocardial conduction.

Allergy is characterized by the typical symptoms of agitation, palpitations, pruritus, coughing, shortness of breath, urticaria, bronchospasm, shock, and convulsions. Treatment measures include administration of oxygen, isotonic intravenous (IV) fluids, intramuscular or subcutaneous adrenaline, and IV prednisolone and aminophylline.

Cardiac effects related to impaired myocardial conduction include bradycardia, cardiac arrest, shock, and convulsions. Emergency treatment measures include the administration of oxygen, IV atropine (0.5 mg) and adrenaline, and the initiation of appropriate cardiac resuscitation. The most common central nervous system manifestations are paresthesia of the tongue, drowsiness, tremor, and convulsions. Options for therapy include IV diazepam and respiratory support.

ACCESS
Adverse Events

The most commonly encountered adverse events related to accessing the endometrial cavity are cervical laceration and perforation of the cervix or the corpus, the latter frequently resulting in premature termination of the procedure. Air embolism, although rare, also may occur at the time of uterine access, and is discussed later.

Background

If the objective lens of the hysteroscope cannot be placed through the cervical canal into the endometrial cavity, hysteroscopic procedures cannot be accomplished. Although dilation of the cervix is frequently not necessary, depending in part on the parity of the woman and the outer diameter of the hysteroscopic system, in some instances active dilation is necessary. In such circumstances, the cervix can be traumatized, possibly leading to lacerations and bleeding that require surgical repair.

Access to the endometrial cavity may be compromised by intrinsic anatomic variation, by acquired anatomic abnormalities of the cervical canal, or by suboptimal technique. Acute version or flexion of the uterus are circumstances that can lead to difficult access. The cervix may also be stenotic relating to a number of factors that include nulliparity, postmenopausal status, and previous surgery such as cesarean section, or previous cervical procedures such as cryotherapy, large-loop excision, or traditional conization. The stenosis may manifest at the level of the exocervix, which is common with, for example, cervices that have been treated with cryotherapy, or at the level of the internal os, which is more common with previous cesarean section. It has also been my experience that access can be made difficult secondary to otherwise asymptomatic Nabothian cysts or leiomyomata that alter the path of the cervical canal.

If dilation of the cervix is required, the most common approach is to use cervical dilators; the tapered semi-rigid O Finder for exocervical stenosis, or rigid standard dilators for stenosis at the level of the internal os. Particularly with rigid dilators, partial or total perforation may result, thereby compromising completion of the procedure.

Even partial perforations may lead to increased systemic absorption of distending media, which is discussed later.

Risk Reduction, Recognition, and Management of Access-related Adverse Events

The risk of complications of access may be largely reduced by any of several pre- or intraoperative measures. If a stenotic cervix is anticipated, there is value in the use of preprocedure techniques to facilitate or initiate cervical dilation. One approach is the use of a natural or synthetic laminaria tent, inserted in the cervix 3 to 8 hours before the procedure. However, positioning of even a thin laminaria requires at least some degree of cervical dilation, all the way through the internal cervical os; a feature that frequently limits the usefulness of this approach. If laminaria are left in place too long in the nonpregnant cervix (eg, longer than 24 hours), the cervix may overdilate, which is particularly counterproductive for CO_2 insufflation.

Another approach, and one that I prefer, is the use of oral or vaginal prostaglandin E_1 (misoprostol) administered 12 to 24 hours before the procedure (400 µg orally or 200 µg vaginally). There is high quality evidence demonstrating efficacy in reducing the need for dilation and the incidence of related cervical trauma when dilation is required.[13,14] Administration too soon before the procedure may result in a suboptimal response, even if used sublingually.[15] Misoprostol may be ineffective as a cervical ripening agent in postmenopausal women,[16] but the addition of systemic estrogen for two weeks before the procedure may provide results similar to those reported for premenopausal patients.[17]

If cervical stenosis is encountered, and misoprostol or laminaria have not been used or were ineffective, deep intracervical injection of dilute vasopressin (0.05 U/mL, 4 mL at 4 and 8 o'clock on the cervix) also substantially reduces the force required for cervical dilation.[18] Care must be taken with the use of vasopressin, particularly in a nonmonitored environment, as systemic injection can result in several cardiorespiratory complications. Consequently, this step should be reserved for hysteroscopy in a setting in which appropriate resuscitative measures can be taken should an adverse reaction occur.

In the procedure or operating room, the surgeon should assess the need for cervical dilation; in many instances, a 3- to 5-mm outside diameter sheath can be passed with no dilation, or using hydrodilation (the pressure exerted by the distending media). Positioning a hysteroscope may be especially useful in the circumstance of a stenotic or tortuous cervical canal because visually directed navigation is preferable to blind and forced dilation that may result in perforation. In the circumstance of previous access failure, we have found that adhesions or synechiae in the canal frequently exist. In such instances, the use of mechanical scissors passed through the operating channel can be used to divide the adhesions under direct vision.

If dilators are required, the process should be completed as atraumatically as possible. It is best to avoid using a uterine sound because it can traumatize the canal or the endometrium, causing unnecessary bleeding and uterine perforation. Difficult cases may be aided using ultrasound guidance, by transabdominal technique with the bladder adequately filled to function as a sonic viewing window. For obese patients, transrectal ultrasound may be preferable.

At the end of the procedure, the cervix should be inspected for laceration and bleeding. Minor bleeding may be managed with tamponade and time, whereas larger tears, or those for which bleeding is not managed successfully by pressure, may require the placement of a delayed absorbable suture.

DISTENDING MEDIA
Adverse Events

Rarely, adverse reactions to selected distending agents can be encountered and gas embolization may, in some instances, be a serious complication. More commonly, and especially with nonphysiologic distending media, fluid and electrolyte disturbances may result from excess systemic absorption.

Background

Distention of the endometrial cavity is necessary to create a viewing space for visual diagnosis and for the performance of surgical procedures. The media choices include CO_2 gas, high-viscosity 32% dextran 70, and several low-viscosity fluids, including nonelectrolytic solutions of glycine, sorbitol, mannitol, and dextrose in water, and electrolyte-containing isotonic solutions such as normal saline. For diagnostic and simple procedures, this is rarely a concern but, during many operative procedures, these agents can gain access to the systemic circulation if the integrity of the uterine venous circulation is breached. In the extreme, fluid overload may occur, and, with the use of nonphysiologic fluids, electrolyte disturbances typically result.

Large volumes of distending media can quickly enter the systemic circulation, particularly when myometrial dissection results in the transection of larger veins. Patients can develop severe hyponatremia, right heart failure, and pulmonary and cerebral edema with resulting death. There is evidence that cerebral edema may be detectable with as little as 500 mL absorption into the systemic circulation.[19,20] Consequently, it is critically important to take measures to reduce the risk of systemic absorption, to monitor the volume of fluid absorbed, and to manage the patient promptly and effectively if excess absorption is suspected or detected.

Calculation of systemic absorption can be complicated by several factors. It can be difficult to capture of all the media that exits the uterus, including that which may fall on the floor of the procedure or operating room. Furthermore, there is inconsistency with the volume of several of the media solutions packaged in large 3-L bags that have a volume that is typically 3% to 6% more than that indicated on the label.[21] The amount of distending media absorbed is also related to the intracavitary pressure; exceeding the mean arterial pressure may facilitate absorption into the systemic circulation.[22]

Issues Related to Type of Distending Media

CO₂

Carbon dioxide gas can be used as a distending medium for diagnostic hysteroscopy. The gas is transmitted to the endometrial cavity via the sheath of the hysteroscopic system that, in turn, is attached to an insufflator specially designed for the procedure, with rubberized or other suitable connective tubing. Although appropriate for diagnostic purposes, CO_2 is unsuitable for operative hysteroscopy and for diagnostic procedures when the patient is bleeding, because there is no effective way to remove blood and other debris from the endometrial cavity. There is high-quality evidence from randomized trials comparing CO_2 with liquid media that demonstrates increased patient discomfort, reduced patient satisfaction, and longer procedural times with the gaseous media.[23,24]

High-viscosity fluids

The most common high-viscosity fluid used for hysteroscopy is 32% dextran 70, usually sold as Hyskon, which is a hyperosmolar fluid. Dextran 70 is most useful for patients who are bleeding in the endometrial cavity, because it does not mix with blood, thereby facilitating visualization in these circumstances. However, dextran 70 can induce an allergic response, coagulopathy, and, if sufficient volumes are infused, vascular overload and heart failure.[25,26] Because dextran is hydrophilic, it can draw 6 times its own volume into the systemic circulation, resulting in fluid overload and electrolyte disturbances. Consequently, the infused volume of this agent should be limited, probably to no more than 300 mL.

Another issue with dextran 70 is that it tends to carmelize on instruments, which must be disassembled and thoroughly cleaned in warm water immediately after each use. Failure to do so may result in irreversible damage to the hysteroscopic system. Because of this, dextran 70 should never be used with flexible endoscopes.

Low-viscosity fluids

The so-called low-viscosity media, which include 3% sorbitol, 1.5% glycine, 5% mannitol, and combined solutions of sorbitol and mannitol, are commonly used when RF electrosurgery is to be performed using monopolar instruments, because they are nonionic, and, therefore, do not disperse current. However, these hypoosmolar, electrolyte-free media can create fluid and electrolyte disturbances if absorbed in excess.[20] The issue may be more important for premenopausal women because the sodium-potassium ATP-ase pump responsible for shunting sodium, and, indirectly, water, out of the cell is inhibited by female sex steroids; an effect that is largely prevented by the administration of gonadotropin-releasing hormone (GnRH) agonists.[27] This circumstance makes hyponatremia a more risky proposition in premenopausal women, at least in those who undergo resectoscopic surgery without the use of GnRH agonists.[28] Several deaths have been associated with the use of glycine or sorbitol at the time of operative hysteroscopic surgery.[29] Hyperammonemia has been reported to be an independent cause of death associated with resectoscopic surgery of the prostate, but this complication is extremely rare and it is not known to be associated with resectoscopic surgery in the uterus. Animal studies suggest that hyperammonemia likely plays a minor role in morbidity and mortality in cases of fluid overload.[30]. Hypoosmolarity and hyponatremia are more likely to induce the greatest degree of morbidity; whether 5% mannitol (osmolality 274 mOsmol/L), by virtue of its near isosmolar composition (normal osmolality 280 mOsmol/L), is a safer choice than 1.5% glycine (200 mOsmol/L) or 3% sorbitol (179 mOsmol/L) has not been determined and it remains only theoretically advantageous.

Normal saline is a useful and safer medium. If there is absorption of a substantial volume of solution, normal saline does not cause electrolyte imbalance and consequently is a good choice for minor procedures performed in the office. The development of bipolar RF instrumentation for hysteroscopic surgery has allowed the application of saline as a distending medium in more advanced and complex procedures.

Media Delivery and Management Systems

Media delivery systems refer to the method whereby the fluid is delivered to the endometrial cavity. There are several media delivery systems, ranging from simple gravity to automated pumps that maintain a preset pressure.

Distending media management systems apply only to fluid media, and are designed to measure the volume of fluid delivered and the amount that leaves the endometrial cavity thereby providing the opportunity to continuously calculate the amount of systemic absorption. This volume can be estimated manually by capturing, measuring, and then subtracting that collected from the volume infused, or it can be continuously calculated using devices that measure the difference between the weights of media infused from that collected.

Media delivery

CO_2 insufflators For instillation of gasseous (CO_2) media, the insufflator must be especially designed for hysteroscopy; the use of laparoscopic insufflators should be absolutely avoided. Such an approach has been associated with massive CO_2 embolism and death, because laparoscopic insufflator flow rates cannot be reliably adjusted to less than 1000 mL/min.

Syringes Large-capacity syringes can be used for office diagnostic procedures, but are most practicable for infusing dextran 70 solution. The syringe can be operated by the surgeon or an assistant and is connected directly to the sheath or attached by connecting tubing.

Gravity-based systems Continuous hydrostatic pressure is effectively achieved by elevating the vehicle containing the distention media above the level of the patient's uterus using an IV pole or other suitable adjustable device. The achieved pressure is the product of the width of the connecting tubing and the elevation; for operative hysteroscopy with 10-mm tubing, intrauterine pressure ranges from 70 to 100 mm Hg when the bag is between 1 and 1.5 m above the uterine cavity.

Pressurized delivery systems The simplest pressurized delivery system can be created by positioning a pressure cuff around the infusion bag. Such an approach does not allow precise control of the pressure, so that, in prolonged cases, or those associated with violation of the myometrium, excessive extravasation could occur, especially if intrauterine pressure is sustained at more than the mean arterial pressure.

Simple pump devices continue to press fluid into the uterine cavity regardless of resistance, whereas the pressure-sensitive pumps reduce the flow rate when the preset level is reached, thereby impeding the efflux of blood and debris and compromising the view, making these the preferred design.[31] Although there is little value to using these systems in the office diagnostic setting, maintenance of a standard intrauterine pressure is essential for prolonged operative interventions.

Measurement of systemic absorption

The most basic mechanism for measurement of systemic media absorption is the manual measurement of inflow and outflow that captures fluid from 3 sources: the resectoscope, the perineal collection drape, and the floor. The variable volume in the media containers and the rapidity of fluid dynamics make this a clumsy and frequently inaccurate methodology that does not provide real-time metrics.[32] It is preferable to use an automated fluid measurement system that takes into account all of the components but which provides continuous measurement of the amount of distending media absorbed into the systemic circulation (**Fig. 1**). These systems compensate for the variable volume in the infusion bags by using weight to calculate infused volume. Complete collection of all fluid escaping or removed from the endometrial cavity ensures that total weight can be subtracted from infused weight, allowing for accurate calculation of systemic absorption.

Risk Reduction, Recognition, and Management of Media-related Adverse Events

Risk reduction of media-related complications begins well before the procedure starts. Recognition of the types of procedures that are prone to excess media absorption is important because several preoperative measures can be taken to reduce risk. For example, diagnostic hysteroscopy and simple procedures that do not involve the

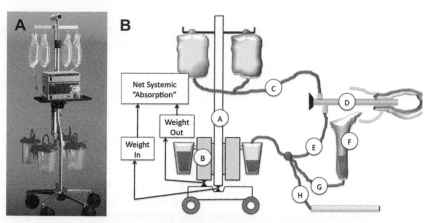

Fig. 1. Automated fluid management systems. (*A*) The system comprises a pump and a mechanism for determining the amount of fluid absorbed by the patient. The pump infuses distending media and controls intrauterine pressure at a setting determined by the surgeon. (*B*) The mechanism of action of the fluid balance component of an automated fluid management system. The infusion media is placed on the pole (A) whereas canisters for collecting evacuated fluid are attached to a separately mounted collection platform (B). The fluid is infused through tubing (C) to the resectoscope (D) that is depicted here passing through the vagina and the cervix into the endometrial cavity. Fluid within the endometrial cavity is evacuated via tubing (E) into the collecting canisters. Fluid that leaks around the resectoscope into the vagina is captured in a specially designed pouch (F), or, if it falls on the floor, by a floor mat, each of which is connected to the collecting canister with tubing (G, H). The pole and the collection platform are independently mounted on devices (generally based on Wheatstone bridges) designed to weigh the fluid electronically. The microprocessor subtracts the collected fluid (Weight Out) from the infused fluid (Weight In) to calculate the fluid balance (the net systemic absorption).

myometrium are low risk for media-related complications. Procedures at higher risk include those that are anticipated to take longer, particularly if they involve dissection in the myometrium such as resection of type I or type II leiomyomas. There is evidence that the risk of fluid overload in resectoscopic myomectomy is directly related to the duration of the procedure, the diameter of the lesion(s), and the proportion of the myoma that is in the myometrium.[33] Recognition of the volume of systemic fluid absorption requires that a media management protocol is in place, and it is preferable that such protocols include the automated fluid management systems described earlier. There should also be predetermined thresholds for the intraoperative measurement of electrolytes, for the use of diuretics, and for expeditious termination of the procedure should excess fluid absorption be detected.

Preoperative
For premenopausal women, the volume of systemically absorbed distension media may be reduced with the preoperative use of GnRH analogs[27,34] and, as discussed earlier, such an approach may lessen the morbidity associated with excess absorption of nonionic hypoosmolar fluid should it occur. Another approach that can be used immediately before cervical dilation is the preoperative administration of dilute vasopressin: 4 mL (total of 8 mL) of dilute intracervical vasopressin (0.01U/mL) injected deeply about 4 and 8 o'clock in the cervix.[35,36] This technique has been shown to reduce the force required for dilation of the cervix.

Gaseous media
Carbon dioxide is highly soluble in blood and, consequently, even if emboli occur, they are rarely clinically significant. These adverse events are discussed later.

Intraoperative fluid media management
Before undertaking a procedure using the resectoscope, baseline serum electrolyte levels should be measured. Women with cardiopulmonary disease should be evaluated carefully for shifts in fluid volume. Absorbed volumes tolerated by healthy women may be catastrophic in the context of compromised cardiac function.

The extent of systemic intravasation can be reduced by operating at the lowest effective intrauterine pressure (50–80 mm Hg), always trying to keep this at less than the mean arterial pressure, and completing the procedure as quickly as possible. There is also evidence that use of bulk vaporizing electrodes is associated with reduced systemic absorption compared with the resection loops, apparently because of the greater degree of electrocoagulation (and resultant collateral vessel sealing) associated with bulk vaporization.[37,38]

Detection of impending excess systemic absorption can prevent fluid overload. Measurement of media infusion and collection should take place in a closed system to allow as precise a calculation as possible of the absorbed volume. If an automated system is not available, the volume should be measured and the deficit calculated every 5 to 10 minutes. Although automated systems are generally unnecessary for diagnostic hysteroscopy and simple procedures such as polypectomy or tubal sterilization, they may be life saving in the context of more advanced resectoscopic procedures such as myomectomy of sizable lesions involving the myometrium.

The management of intraoperatively recognized excessive intravasation varies according to the patient's baseline medical condition, her intraoperative assessment, the status of the procedure, and the amount of measured fluid intravasation. If the deficit reaches a predetermined limit (which, depending on the patient's baseline status, could be 750–1500 mL), serum electrolytes are measured and furosemide is given intravenously, in a dose of 10 to 40 mg, depending on renal function. Should the serum sodium decrease to less than 125 mEq/L, or should the deficit reach 1500 to 2000 mL, the procedure is expeditiously terminated.

Postoperative management of clinically significant fluid and electrolyte disturbances should involve the support of a consultant with expertise in critical care. Patients may manifest with one or a combination of cerebral edema, pulmonary edema, and right heart failure and could require ventilatory support, the use of diuretics and inotropic agents, and the judicious administration of hypertonic saline solutions.

GAS EMBOLI
Adverse Events

Rarely, catastrophic outcomes, including death, have been ascribed to venous gas emboli. In most instances, these emboli are derived from room air, but such emboli may be caused by gaseous distension media or the products of electrosurgical vaporization.

Background

During intrauterine surgical procedures, large uterine veins may be broached, providing an entry point for gaseous substances into the venous systemic circulation if the pressure head of the gas exceeds that in the vein. The gas may gain access to the vena cava then travel to the right heart, the pulmonary arteries, and then to the lungs. If the embolized gas is of sufficient volume, it may interfere with gaseous exchange and cause cardiac arrhythmias, pulmonary hypertension, and, ultimately, decreased pulmonary venous return and reduced cardiac output. When gas embolism occurs in association with a uterine surgical procedure such as Cesarean section,[39] room air seems to be the obvious origin of the embolic material. However, during hysteroscopy, there are several gaseous substances that could gain access to the venous circulation and, in some instances, contribute to cardiovascular compromise and even death.[40–45] Room air is not soluble in blood, and a volume as low as 50 mL may be fatal.[46] However, CO_2 is the gaseous distending medium used for diagnostic hysteroscopy, and is extremely soluble in blood; a characteristic that is responsible for its relative safety. However, should large volumes of CO_2 enter the systemic circulation, serious intraoperative morbidity, and even death, may result.[47–49]

Gaseous emboli may occur without symptoms or adverse clinical events and they may be virtually ubiquitous in resectoscopic surgery in the uterus.[50] The recognition that the products of electrosurgical vaporization may enter the systemic circulation engendered our evaluation of the components of the gases generated by monopolar and bipolar electrosurgical instruments. We were able to determine that the volume of gas produced by these instruments was similar, and that the gaseous products of vaporization largely comprised hydrogen, CO, and CO_2, all of which are rapidly soluble in blood.[51,52] This information suggests that the frequently encountered gas emboli that seem to be the products of tissue vaporization are rapidly dissolved in blood, and rarely, if ever, attain a volume that has clinical significance. Room air largely comprises nitrogen and oxygen, and is less soluble in blood, thereby presenting a greater risk to the cardiovascular integrity of the surgical patient.

During hysteroscopy, air can be introduced into the endometrial cavity via the fluid or gas delivery system, or via the cervix, perhaps aided by factors such as the introduction (and reintroduction) of dilators or hysteroscopic instruments that may function like a piston. If the patient is in the Trendelenberg position, the pressure differential between the endometrial cavity and the right heart increases, thereby facilitating the passage of air that may be present in the endometrial cavity into the uterine veins and the systemic venous circulation.

Recognition, Management, and Risk Reduction

The awake patient experiencing an air embolus will often report dyspnea or chest pain, and there may be symptoms and signs of acute bronchospasm and pulmonary edema. The anesthetized patient will not have symptoms, making intraoperative monitoring the principle method of diagnosis. The most sensitive, but nonspecific, diagnostic test is measurement of end-tidal CO_2, which may signify air embolism with a reduction of as little as 2 mm Hg. However, if pulse oximetry is used, a substantial number will have reduced oxygen saturation,[53,54] and, if found together with reduced end-tidal CO_2, will be suggestive of air embolism. Although there are several nonspecific electrocardiographic changes, including premature ventricular contractions, heart block, and ST-segment depression, a more specific finding is the detection of air in the right heart by precordial auscultation, preferably with Doppler ultrasound seeking the typical millwheel murmur. Transesophageal echocardiography is more sensitive, but the technique is not routinely used during hysteroscopic procedures because of its expense, technical demands, and invasive nature.[45]

If air embolism (or clinically significant gas embolism) is suspected, the point of suspected air entry should be identified and closed, which generally means removing any instruments from the uterus and clamping closed the cervical canal. The patient should be placed in the Trendelenberg position, and rolled onto the left side (Durant maneuver), an orientation that may reduce the risk of air occluding the outflow tract by placing the right ventricle more superiorly.[55] The administration of 100% oxygen should be initiated, and a central venous catheter or direct needle puncture of the right heart should be used to identify and remove the air or other gas.[56] Cardiopulmonary resuscitation and inotropic support are frequently necessary.

Risk reduction starts with education of the staff included in the procedure, especially the surgeon and the anesthesiologist, if one is participating in the case. Measures should be taken to minimize the effort needed to dilate the cervix because many emboli are related to the process of access, discussed elsewhere in this article. It is best to avoid placing the patient in the Trendelenberg position because of the potential for increasing the pressure head in the endometrial cavity compared with the right heart.

Reducing the risk of clinically significant CO_2 emboli requires that the surgeon use only an insufflator specifically designed for hysteroscopy because, for example, even the lowest settings on laparoscopic insufflators would pump dangerous volumes of gas into the endometrial cavity. Ensuring that the insufflation pressure is less than 100 mm Hg and the flow rate less than 100 mL/min can essentially eliminate these risks. As discussed earlier, CO_2 should be avoided if operative procedures are performed.

The process of reducing the risk of air emboli is clearly multifactorial. Before inserting the hysteroscopic system into the endometrial cavity, the tubing and hysteroscope should be purged of air even if the distention medium is CO_2. The number of instrument exchanges should be minimized because, for example, each removal and reinsertion of the resectoscope provides an additional opportunity for the pistonlike action of the hysteroscope assembly to push air into the systemic circulation. Leaving the cervical canal open to the atmosphere may facilitate the access of air to the systemic circulation, so a dilator or other occlusive instrument should always be left in the canal following the process of dilation.

PERFORATION
Adverse Events

Although complete uterine perforation usually results in an inability to maintain a distended uterus, thereby resulting in premature termination of the procedure, the serious consequences of perforation relate to damage to surrounding viscera and blood vessels.

Background

Perforation of the uterus may be partial or complete. In most instances, the perforation occurs during sounding or dilation of the cervix, but the complication may be a result of the hysteroscopic or resectoscopic procedure itself. Complete perforations are generally believed to result in inability to distend the endometrial cavity, or, if the injury occurs following establishment of a working space, by otherwise inexplicable loss of distension. In either instance, the surgeon is generally unable to continue the procedure.

When complete perforation occurs as a result of dilation of the cervix, there are usually no other injuries. However, should the uterus be perforated by a sharp hysteroscopic instrument or with the activated the tip of a laser or an RF electrode, there is a risk for injury to the adjacent blood vessels or viscera. Without further measures, such injuries are frequently complicated by delayed diagnosis, which is a particular problem for small bowel injury, from which mortality is high.[57,58]

Prevention, Recognition, and Management

Because most perforations occur at the time of dilation of the cervix, it is important to reduce risk by taking the steps described earlier.

When using a resectoscope, the general rule is that the operator should not advance the electrode while it is activated. Such an approach should essentially eliminate perforation with electrosurgically induced damage to large blood vessels and the viscera that surround the uterus in the pelvis, including bowel, ureter, and bladder. The exceptions to this rule are the division of a uterine septum and bulk vaporization of myomas, particularly when they are in fundal locations. Consequently, perhaps a more tenable rule would be to avoid any forward movement of an activated electrode while in the endometrium or myometrium.

An area susceptible to perforation is the uterine cornu where myometrial thickness may be as little as 4 mm. Consequently, the surgeon should be extremely careful when performing resection in this region. If resectoscopic endometrial ablation is being performed, it may be best to use careful rollerball-based electrosurgical desiccation in this region.

In select cases, there may value in performing simultaneous ultrasound or laparoscopy to reduce the risk of perforation or injury to surrounding viscera and blood vessels. Transabdominal ultrasound, in most instances, allows for visualization of the endometrial cavity distended with the sololucent contrasting fluid media, as well as the myometrium and the surrounding echogenic serosal surface (**Fig. 2**). Within this fluid-filled space, the hysteroscope and, if appropriately aligned, the electrode or scissors can usually be seen, a view that allows the surgeon to reduce the risk of perforation. This approach may be useful for selected metroplasties, when performing myomectomy on deep type 1 or type 2 lesions, or for directing adhesiolysis in cases of Asherman syndrome when the usual intracavitary landmarks may be obscured.

Simultaneous laparoscopy does not provide the same value in preventing perforation, but it can ensure that bowel or bladder is not attached or adjacent to the area of dissection, usually simply by virtue of the intraperitoneal gas and laparoscopically directed positioning of the uterus. This approach may be of particular value when performing laparoscopy in circumstances in which perforation is a substantial risk and transabdominal ultrasound is not available or successful because of body habitus or uterine configuration or orientation. There is also value in the context of previous uterine surgery, such as laparoscopic or laparotomic myomectomy, when adhesions to the uterine serosa could place bowel at increased risk for injury.

If a perforation has occurred and there is evidence of bleeding or presumed visceral injury (especially with the activated tip or a laser or electrosurgical electrode), laparoscopy or laparotomy should be performed. Injury to the uterus is usually easy to detect with a laparoscope. However, mechanical or thermal injury to the bowel, ureter, or bladder is more difficult and may require laparotomy for complete assessment. If the patient's condition is managed expectantly, overnight admission should be considered, and she should be asked to report any symptoms of visceral trauma such as fever, increasing pain, nausea, and vomiting. Thermal injury to the intestine or ureter may be difficult to diagnose, and symptoms may not occur for several days to two weeks. Further management of these injuries is beyond the scope of this article.

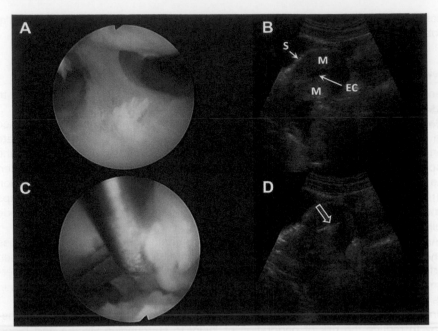

Fig. 2. Ultrasound-guided intrauterine surgery. Transabdominal ultrasound can be used, in combination with hysteroscopy, to reduce the risk of perforation. Intrauterine adhesions are seen hysteroscopically (*A*) and the simultaneous transabdominal image is shown (*B*) with the well-defined endometrial cavity (EC), myometrium (M), and uterine serosa (S). The 5 French mechanical scissors are shown hysteroscopically (*C*) and their echogenic image (*arrow*) is easily visualized (*D*).

BLEEDING
Adverse Events

Intraoperative bleeding may emanate from the endometrium, myometrium, or from damage to periuterine vessels. In most instances, this bleeding will be recognized intraoperatively, but, in some cases, presentation will be delayed for several hours.

Background

The uterus is endowed with a rich blood supply that originates from the uterine and ovarian arteries, with the largest-caliber myometrial vessels increasing in diameter from the endometrial to serosal surfaces.

The uterine artery originates from the internal iliac artery then bifurcates, usually near the uterine isthmus within the broad ligament, resulting in a descending cervical branch and an ascending branch that anastamoses with the ovarian artery near the fundus. As the ascending branches course cephalad, they give rise to 6 to 10 arcuate arteries posteriorly and anteriorly, each of which anastamose with corresponding vessels from the contralateral side, thereby forming a stacked series of vascular rings. The myometrium receives its blood supply from centrifugal and centripetally oriented branches of the arcuate arteries that are oriented in a radial fashion, perpendicular to the serosal surface. When the centripetally oriented radial arteries cross the endomyometrial junction, they give rise to the smaller-caliber basal arteries, but continue toward the endometrial surface as the spiral arteries that provide blood supply to the functionalis layer of endometrium. Bleeding that occurs during or after operative hysteroscopic procedures, especially resectoscopic surgery, generally results from trauma to the myometrial vessels or, if uterine perforation occurs, injury to uterine arteries or other vessels in the pelvis.

Prevention, Recognition, and Management

Anemic patients, who have low tolerance for intraoperative blood loss, can be rendered amenorrheic before surgery with GnRH analogs and provided iron therapy, thereby increasing their preoperative hemoglobin and iron stores. If such a surgical delay is not feasible, preoperative blood transfusion can be considered. Another consideration, particularly when planning operations that involve deep resection, is the preoperative collection and storage of autologous blood.

Although rare, arteriovenous (AV) malformations may be confused with leiomyomas and, should resection be attempted on such a vascular lesion, massive bleeding may ensue. Consequently, should there be any suspicion that a focal lesion involving the myometrium is an AV malformation, preoperative assessment with Doppler ultrasound or magnetic resonance imaging is advised.

The risk or extent of intraoperative bleeding may also be reduced by preoperatively administered GnRH analogs or the intraoperative (just before cervical dilation) injection of diluted vasopressin into the cervical stroma in the same concentrations, doses, and techniques described previously to reduce the force of dilation.[36] The duration of action of dilute vasopressin is about 20 minutes, so repeat dosing may be of value. It is important to avoid intravascular injection and to advise the anesthesiologist in advance of such injections to facilitate recognition of rare, but important, adverse events such as hypertension and bronchospasm.

The risk for injury to the larger-caliber myometrial branches of the uterine artery can be reduced by limiting the depth of resection in the lateral endometrial cavity near the uterine isthmus, where RF vaporization or electrodesiccation techniques should be considered.

When intracavitary bleeding is encountered during resectoscopic procedures, temporary increase of the intrauterine pressure may reduce the blood flow sufficiently to improve visualization and allow targeting of a large-caliber ball electrode for compression, then electrosurgical desiccation. Intractable bleeding may respond to the injection of diluted vasopressin deep into the cervical stroma, again in doses and techniques described previously. Another approach to the management of intracavitary bleeding recognized at the end of a procedure (often secondary to the loss of intrauterine tamponade effect from the distending media) is the inflation of a 30-mL Foley catheter balloon or similar device.[59] Such balloons can easily be inflated to 50 mL if necessary.

Management of suspected intraperitoneal bleeding, the result of perforation of the uterus, will require laparoscopic evaluation or laparotomy, depending on the clinical situation. The management of injury to major vessels is beyond the scope of this article.

ELECTROSURGERY
Adverse Events

Thermal injury can occur to intraperitoneal structures, especially bowel, if an activated electrode perforates the myometrium and serosal surface. Such an injury could occur without perforation if bowel was adherent to the serosal surface and deep myometrial electrosurgical techniques were used. Injury may also occur at the site of placement of the dispersive electrode if it is improperly placed or dislodged. Rarely, with monopolar instrumentation, current diversion may occur, causing injury to one or a combination of the cervix, vagina, or vulva.

Background

Principles of RF electrosurgery

Electrosurgery is the application of RF alternating current to increase intracellular temperature, resulting in tissue vaporization or the combination of desiccation and coagulation. The incumbent requirement to apply energy in a fluid environment presents several challenges to surgeons and to the manufacturers of hysteroscopic surgical equipment. The surgeon should be familiar with electrical principles as they apply to the equipment, thus ensuring that the desired tissue effect is achieved and risks of complications are minimized.

RF electrosurgery requires the creation of a circuit for the passage of electrons that includes two electrodes, the patient, the electrosurgical generator or unit (ESU) and the connecting wires. All RF electrosurgical systems require two electrodes, a feature that makes all electrosurgery, in effect, bipolar. Monopolar instruments have only an active electrode for concentrating and delivering the current to the target tissue, whereas the second large electrode is attached remotely on the patient. Although this electrode is often called a return electrode, the appropriate name is the dispersive electrode because it defocuses or diffuses the current at the contact point, thereby preventing a local tissue effect. Monopolar instrumentation is designed so the entire patient is involved in the circuit, a circumstance that provides a greater opportunity for current to be diverted to undesirable locations.

Bipolar instruments are designed to contain both electrodes. This circumstance limits the portion of the patient involved in the circuit to the tissue that is near to, or interposed between, the two electrodes. Most bipolar instruments are designed to have two active electrodes, such as is the case for laparoscopic sealing forceps, but, for bipolar hysteroscopic systems, the second electrode's function is dispersive.

When the RF electromagnetic energy is applied to tissue, it is first converted to intracellular mechanical energy, manifesting in oscillation of intracellular proteins, then, as a result of the frictional forces generated from these rapidly moving molecules, the mechanical energy is transformed to thermal energy. If the energy is focused and the cell is heated rapidly, beyond the boiling point of water (100°C), the cellular water turns to steam, rapidly and massively expanding the intracellular volume, which quickly results in cell rupture; a process called vaporization. If the intracellular temperature is sharply increased to more than 60°C, but remains less than the boiling point of water, the intracellular water is lost by the process of dehydration or desiccation. Simultaneously, the molecular bonds of collagenous tissue are hyperthermally broken then haphazardly reformed when the tissue cools, creating a homogenous coagulum in a process called coagulation. The type of tissue effect is generally determined by the area of the electrode-tissue interface, the most important factor in determining current density, but is also importantly related to the waveform and the voltage and current output of the generator, the product of which is expressed in watts.

Electrosurgery in the uterus

The intrauterine environment presents the challenge of establishing and maintaining the RF tissue effects in the context of a fluid medium. Because electrolyte-containing distention media such as saline are effective conductors, they disperse the current from the active electrode of a monopolar instrument, preventing the creation of the zone of high current density necessary to achieve the desired electrosurgical tissue effect. Consequently, for monopolar instrumentation, it is necessary to use electrolyte-free distention media, such as sorbitol, glycine, or mannitol, that are electrolyte free and, therefore, nonconductive, and, in this case, nondispersive.

Bipolar resectoscopic instruments are generally designed with a distal active electrode and a more proximal dispersive electrode, a configuration that allows for the completion of a circuit in an electrolyte-rich medium like normal saline. Compared with monopolar systems, the distance between the two electrodes is greatly decreased, reducing circuit impedance, and, with ionic oscillation, formation of a steam envelope and completion of the circuit as the ESU is activated. Despite these features, there are several design and construction issues that make bipolar resectoscopes less efficient than monopolar versions, a feature that makes many surgeons reluctant to switch despite the inherent safety provided by being able to work in normal-saline distending media.

Monopolar and bipolar instruments, when used to vaporize tissue, produce the same vapor cloud that, in fluid media, manifests as an array of bubbles that largely consist of hydrogen, CO, and CO_2, each of which is highly soluble in blood.[51] Consequently, should these products enter the systemic circulation (as they often do), they rapidly dissolve in blood and do not present a cause for concern for the patient.

Resectoscopic RF complications

Active electrode injury Active electrode injury can occur with monopolar and bipolar instruments. Perhaps the most common active electrode injury is secondary to inadvertent activation of the ESU when the resectoscope is in contact with the patient's skin, the vulva, or the vagina. The other injuries largely relate to perforation with an activated electrode that can subsequently injure bowel, bladder, or other intraperitoneal structures, including blood vessels. Bleeding may present acutely, but injury to bowel or bladder, and subsequent peritonitis, may not manifest for several days, a circumstance that can have disastrous consequences for the patient.

Current diversion Unique to monopolar resectoscopes is the complication of current diversion, which can result in injury to the cervix, vagina, or vulva. Understanding the mechanisms involved in such complications is the key to reducing the risk of occurrence.

Monopolar uterine resectoscopes allow transfer of RF energy from the active electrode to the external sheath by direct contact (direct coupling) or without contact (capacitative coupling), the latter being related to the energy field around any circuit. Regardless of the amount of energy so transmitted, provided there is an intimate contact between the external sheath and the surrounding cervix, the diverted circuit will be completed between the active and dispersive electrodes without the creation of an area of high current density where an undesirable burn could occur. However, if the intimate relationship of the external sheath with the cervix is lost, the current can be diverted to another path, which could result in a zone of high current density on the vagina or vulva (**Fig. 3**).[60] These are the presumed mechanisms for a growing series of vulvar and vaginal thermal injuries reported in conjunction with the use of monopolar uterine resectoscopes.[61]

The most obvious cause of direct coupling is a breech in the electrode's insulation that, when appropriately flexed, results in contact with the internal sheath or telescope, with capacitative coupling (the transfer of energy from one otherwise unconnected circuit to another by means of mutual capacitance) completing the circuit with the external sheath. However, another potential mechanism of direct coupling is the existence of tissue fragments, the result of resection, that bridge the gap between the active electrode and internal or external sheaths.[62] The risk of

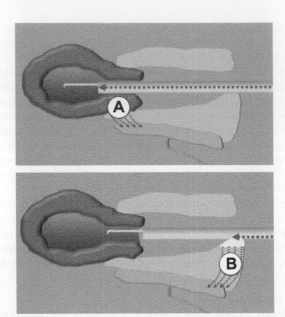

Fig. 3. Current diversion and vulvar vaginal burns. A probable mechanism for vulvar and vaginal burns. (*A, top*) The external sheath contacts the entire surface of the cervical canal. Current between the generator and the electrode (*hatched line*) that capacitatively couples to the external sheath is prevented from forming a zone of high current density as it completes the circuit with the dispersive electrode. (*B*) The external sheath has been removed, preventing contact of the external sheath with the surface of the cervical canal. In this situation, current coupled with the sheath will complete the circuit via the contact with the vagina, which, if of sufficiently low surface area, will allow generation of a zone of high current density that can create an undesired electrosurgical effect.

capacitative coupling seems to be increased with the use of high-voltage currents such as those that come from the coagulation side of ESUs.[63] Capacitative coupling is also more likely to occur if the surgeon keeps the electrode continuously active while not in direct or near contact with tissue, or when there are continuing attempts to desiccate already-desiccated tissue.

Probably the key mechanism in the generation of vulvar and vaginal thermal injuries is loss of contact between the external sheath and the cervix. The most likely explanations are some combination of overdilation or externalization of the external sheath, a circumstance that may occur more often when the cervical canal is short or when the surgeon functions by withdrawing the entire sheath while keeping the activated electrode fully extended.[60]

Risk Minimization, Recognition, and Management

The following principles serve to reduce the risk of electrosurgical injuries. First and foremost, the pedals controlling the electrode should not be placed in a location that facilitates inadvertent activation, and it may be wise to leave the ESU in standby mode until the resectoscope is within the endometrial cavity.

One choice that can be made is to operate using a bipolar resectoscope, because with these instruments there is no opportunity for current diversion and, as discussed earlier, the issue of electrolyte disturbances becomes moot. However, many do not have access to such instrumentation, or, if they do, the efficiency of monopolar systems makes them the preferred devices. Consequently, this discussion refers only to monopolar instruments.

The dispersive electrode (monopolar resectoscopes only) should be securely affixed to the patient, usually on the thigh, in a location that is not disrupted by previous surgery or trauma, such as a previous graft or burn site. Most current generators possess an impedance-based safety mechanism to ensure that the dispersive electrode is attached to the generator and to detect inadequate attachment to the patient, but older ESUs may not have this important safeguard. As described earlier, advancement of an activated electrode should be avoided in the myometrium. Even in selected instances, such as metroplasty or bulk vaporization of a leiomyoma, the electrode should never be advanced unless it can be easily seen and the relationship between the electrode and the uterine serosa is clear.

The use of electrodes with damaged insulation should be avoided. A new electrode should be used for each case. It is probably safer to use low-voltage ("cutting") current, minimizing or avoiding the use of high-voltage ("coagulation") outputs, because such waveforms probably facilitate these complications. Even with resectoscopic electrodesiccation, it is apparent that low- and high-voltage outputs are equivalent with respect to clinical outcome.[64] More importantly, the surgeon should strive to maintain intimate contact between the external sheath and the cervix by not overdilating before starting the procedure and by keeping the external sheath fully in the cervix when operating. The electrode should be activated only when near to, or in contact with, the target tissue, and the temptation to overdesiccate tissue should be avoided.

One sign of current diversion is the absence or reduction of the electrosurgical effect. Following determination that power to the ESU and connections in the circuit are intact, the temptation is often to increase the generator output. Care should be taken to ensure that potentially traumatic current diversion is not taking place.

Any metallic object, such as a vaginal speculum or a cervical tenaculum, also can, following contact with the external sheath, serve to conduct current to locations in the vagina and vulva. Care should be taken to avoid contact of these instruments with the resectoscope.

INFECTION
Problems

Postoperative endomyometritis
Infection of the endometrium or myometrium following hysteroscopic procedures is rarely encountered.

Background

Despite hysteroscopy being performed through the contaminated environment of the vagina, the reported rate of endomyometritis ranges from 0.01% to 1.42%.[3,65] There is some evidence that infection is more common following adhesiolysis on uterine synechiae[65] or when resectoscopic surgery is performed on women with a history of pelvic inflammatory disease (PID).[66]

Risk Reduction, Recognition, and Management

The low frequency of infection in the average patient makes it difficult to design a study with sufficient sample size to determine the value of prophylactic antibiotics. Consequently, studies with surrogate outcomes have been devised, such as a randomized trial evaluating bacteremia in patients receiving prophylactic IV amoxicillin-clavulanate.[67] However, the investigators were unable to show that the prophylactic antibiotics resulted in a reduction in the incidence of clinically significant bacteremia. A Cochrane systematic review was unable to come to any conclusions regarding prophylactic antibiotics because there were no available randomized trials with clinically relevant outcomes.[68] As a result, the American College of Obstetricians and Gynecologists' guidelines do not recommend routine prophylactic antibiotics for hysteroscopic procedures, instead suggesting selective prophylaxis for women with a history of PID.[69]

Endomyometritis may present in the days following the hysteroscopic procedure with some combination of pain, odorous discharge, fever, and tenderness on manual examination of the uterus. The white count may be increased with a left shift. Data regarding the microflora to be expected as causative organisms are sparse. Consequently, the selection of antibiotics and their route of administration are based on the clinical circumstances, including the patient's preexisting medical status and the presumed severity of the infection. For the patient who is medically fit, with few findings, and who is able to tolerate oral medications, cephalosporins or extended-spectrum penicillins will likely suffice, with appropriate follow-up in 48 to 72 hours to ensure that the patient is experiencing an acceptable clinical response. Patients with significant comorbidities, who cannot tolerate, or do not respond to oral antibiotics, or who show evidence of more severe infection, including pelvic sepsis, will likely require hospital admission and the use of parenteral antibiotics, using single agents or multidrug therapy, as appropriate.

LATE COMPLICATIONS
Problems

There are several potential late-onset sequelae of hysteroscopic surgery that may manifest as a result of adhesions within the cervical canal or endometrial cavity. Defects in the integrity of the myometrium may leave the uterus susceptible to rupture in a subsequent pregnancy. Pregnancy following endometrial ablation is almost always an undesired outcome and can be associated with an increased incidence of complications.

Background

Surgery within the uterus can result in the development of adhesions that can have a variety of consequences. Hematometria can develop following endometrial resection if cervical stenosis occludes the outflow of blood from the endometrial cavity. Another entity, called post-tubal occlusion for permanent contraception endometrial ablation syndrome, has been described to occur in the context of an endometrial ablation performed in a woman who has had a previous tubal occlusion for permanent contraception. Synechiae within the endometrial cavity can prevent efflux of blood through the cervix, whereas the occluded tubes prevent passage of blood into the peritoneal cavity, resulting in cyclic pain associated with endometrial bleeding.[70] It is not clear whether such a syndrome could follow transcervical sterilization with devices such as Essure or Adiana.

Several hysteroscopic procedures are designed to treat infertility or recurrent pregnancy loss, or to manage abnormal uterine bleeding while maintaining fertility. In the event of a pregnancy, uterine rupture is a potential consequence, particularly if the hysteroscopic surgery violated the integrity of the myometrium. One review of the literature involving pregnancy-associated uterine rupture after hysteroscopic surgery identified 12 of 14 cases that had occurred following hysteroscopic metroplasty.[71]

Intraoperative perforation had been reported with most of these cases, and most procedures were performed using intrauterine electrosurgery.

Endometrial ablation can never be considered to be a global therapy. As a result, pregnancy can result in women in the reproductive years, of whom only the minority have an uncomplicated course, at least according to a review of 74 reported cases collated and published in 2006.[72] Disorders of placental implantation have been reported including placenta accreta and increta, and a case of uterine rupture resulted in a maternal death.[73,74]

Risk Reduction

Women who choose to undergo endometrial ablation should be strongly cautioned regarding possible longer-term adverse events. Continuing with an effective contraceptive method until menopause or whenever the risk of pregnancy is determined to be over can largely prevent the complications associated with gestation and previous endometrial ablation. Should a pregnancy ensue in such a woman, she should be appropriately counseled regarding the risks of continuing the pregnancy, and, should the pregnancy continue and reach viability, appropriate investigation and planning should surround the delivery.

For women who have already had a sterilization procedure, at least those with ligation, clips, rings or electrodesiccation, counseling before endometrial ablation should include the possibility that cyclic pain may be a longer-term adverse event.

When intrauterine surgery is performed to preserve or enhance fertility, there may be value in a second-look hysteroscopic procedure 4 to 8 weeks following the index procedure. At that time, residual adhesions can be easily lysed with hysteroscopic scissors or even with the tip of the hysteroscope. If there are concerns regarding the integrity of the myometrium, hysteroscopy can be combined with infusion sonography to evaluate the thickness of the myometrium. This approach may facilitate counseling regarding the risk of uterine rupture should a pregnancy ensue. In any instance in which there has been substantial dissection in the myometrium, the patient and her obstetrician should be counseled that uterine rupture is a real risk of subsequent pregnancy. It may be wise to deliver as soon as lung maturity is reached and to consider Cesarean section as a primary delivery method.

REFERENCES

1. Pantaleone DC. On endoscopic examination of the cavity of the womb. Medical Press and Circular London 1869;8:26–7.
2. Jansen FW, Vredevoogd CB, van Ulzen K, et al. Complications of hysteroscopy: a prospective, multicenter study. Obstet Gynecol 2000;96(2):266–70.
3. Aydeniz B, Gruber IV, Schauf B, et al. A multicenter survey of complications associated with 21,676 operative hysteroscopies. Eur J Obstet Gynecol Reprod Biol 2002;104(2):160–4.
4. Propst AM, Liberman RF, Harlow BL, et al. Complications of hysteroscopic surgery: predicting patients at risk. Obstet Gynecol 2000;96(4):517–20.
5. Overton C, Hargreaves J, Maresh M. A national survey of the complications of endometrial destruction for menstrual disorders: the MISTLETOE study. Br J Obstet Gynaecol 1997;104(12):1351–9.
6. Dua RS, Bankes MJ, Dowd GS, et al. Compartment syndrome following pelvic surgery in the lithotomy position. Ann R Coll Surg Engl 2002;84(3):170–1.
7. Cohen SA, Hurt WG. Compartment syndrome associated with lithotomy position and intermittent compression stockings. Obstet Gynecol 2001;97(5 Pt 2):832–3.

8. Meyer RS, White KK, Smith JM, et al. Intramuscular and blood pressures in legs positioned in the hemilithotomy position: clarification of risk factors for well-leg acute compartment syndrome. J Bone Joint Surg Am 2002;84(10):1829–35.
9. Irvin W, Andersen W, Taylor P, et al. Minimizing the risk of neurologic injury in gynecologic surgery. Obstet Gynecol 2004;103(2):374–82.
10. Hopper CL, Baker JB. Bilateral femoral neuropathy complicating vaginal hysterectomy. Analysis of contributing factors in 3 patients. Obstet Gynecol 1968;32(4): 543–7.
11. Burkhart FL, Daly JW. Sciatic and peroneal nerve injury: a complication of vaginal operations. Obstet Gynecol 1966;28(1):99–102.
12. Erickson TB, Kirkpatrick DH, DeFrancesco MS, et al. Executive summary of the American College of Obstetricians and Gynecologists Presidential Task Force on patient safety in the office setting: reinvigorating safety in office-based gynecologic surgery. Obstet Gynecol 2010;115(1):147–51.
13. Thomas JA, Leyland N, Durand N, et al. The use of oral misoprostol as a cervical ripening agent in operative hysteroscopy: a double-blind, placebo-controlled trial. Am J Obstet Gynecol 2002;186(5):876–9.
14. Preutthipan S, Herabutya Y. Vaginal misoprostol for cervical priming before operative hysteroscopy: a randomized controlled trial. Obstet Gynecol 2000;96(6): 890–4.
15. Mulayim B, Celik NY, Onalan G, et al. Sublingual misoprostol for cervical ripening before diagnostic hysteroscopy in premenopausal women: a randomized, double blind, placebo-controlled trial. Fertil Steril 2010;93(7):2400–4.
16. Oppegaard KS, Nesheim BI, Istre O, et al. Comparison of self-administered vaginal misoprostol versus placebo for cervical ripening prior to operative hysteroscopy using a sequential trial design. BJOG 2008;115(5):663, e661–9.
17. Oppegaard KS, Lieng M, Berg A, et al. A combination of misoprostol and estradiol for preoperative cervical ripening in postmenopausal women: a randomised controlled trial. BJOG 2010;117(1):53–61.
18. Phillips DR, Nathanson HG, Milim SJ, et al. The effect of dilute vasopressin solution on the force needed for cervical dilatation: a randomized controlled trial. Obstet Gynecol 1997;89(4):507–11.
19. Istre O, Skajaa K, Schjoensby AP, et al. Changes in serum electrolytes after transcervical resection of endometrium and submucous fibroids with use of glycine 1.5% for uterine irrigation. Obstet Gynecol 1992;80(2):218–22.
20. Istre O, Bjoennes J, Naess R, et al. Postoperative cerebral oedema after transcervical endometrial resection and uterine irrigation with 1.5% glycine. Lancet 1994; 344(8931):1187–9.
21. Nezhat CH, Fisher DT, Datta S. Investigation of often-reported ten percent hysteroscopy fluid overfill: is this accurate? J Minim Invasive Gynecol 2007;14(4): 489–93.
22. Bennett KL, Ohrmundt C, Maloni JA. Preventing intravasation in women undergoing hysteroscopic procedures. AORN J 1996;64(5):792–9.
23. Pellicano M, Guida M, Zullo F, et al. Carbon dioxide versus normal saline as a uterine distension medium for diagnostic vaginoscopic hysteroscopy in infertile patients: a prospective, randomized, multicenter study. Fertil Steril 2003;79(2): 418–21.
24. Brusco GF, Arena S, Angelini A. Use of carbon dioxide versus normal saline for diagnostic hysteroscopy. Fertil Steril 2003;79(4):993–7.
25. Golan A, Siedner M, Bahar M, et al. High-output left ventricular failure after dextran use in an operative hysteroscopy. Fertil Steril 1990;54(5):939–41.

26. Choban MJ, Kalhan SB, Anderson RJ, et al. Pulmonary edema and coagulopathy following intrauterine instillation of 32% dextran-70 (Hyskon). J Clin Anesth 1991; 3(4):317–9.
27. Taskin O, Buhur A, Birincioglu M, et al. Endometrial Na+, K+-ATPase pump function and vasopressin levels during hysteroscopic surgery in patients pretreated with GnRH agonist. J Am Assoc Gynecol Laparosc 1998;5(2):119–24.
28. Ayus JC, Wheeler JM, Arieff AI. Postoperative hyponatremic encephalopathy in menstruant women. Ann Intern Med 1992;117(11):891–7.
29. Baggish MS, Brill AI, Rosenweig B, et al. Fatal acute glycine and sorbitol toxicity during operative hysteroscopy. J Gynecol Surg 1998;9:137–43.
30. Bernstein GT, Loughlin KR, Gittes RF. The physiologic basis of the TUR syndrome. J Surg Res 1989;46(2):135–41.
31. Shirk GJ, Gimpelson RJ. Control of intrauterine fluid pressure during operative hysteroscopy. J Am Assoc Gynecol Laparosc 1994;1(3):229–33.
32. Boyd HR, Stanley C. Sources of error when tracking irrigation fluids during hysteroscopic procedures. J Am Assoc Gynecol Laparosc 2000;7(4):472–6.
33. Emanuel MH, Hart A, Wamsteker K, et al. An analysis of fluid loss during transcervical resection of submucous myomas. Fertil Steril 1997;68(5):881–6.
34. Donnez J, Vilos G, Gannon MJ, et al. Goserelin acetate (Zoladex) plus endometrial ablation for dysfunctional uterine bleeding: a large randomized, double-blind study. Fertil Steril 1997;68(1):29–36.
35. Goldenberg M, Zolti M, Bider D, et al. The effect of intracervical vasopressin on the systemic absorption of glycine during hysteroscopic endometrial ablation. Obstet Gynecol 1996;87(6):1025–9.
36. Phillips DR, Nathanson HG, Milim SJ, et al. The effect of dilute vasopressin solution on blood loss during operative hysteroscopy: a randomized controlled trial. Obstet Gynecol 1996;88(5):761–6.
37. Vercellini P, Oldani S, Yaylayan L, et al. Randomized comparison of vaporizing electrode and cutting loop for endometrial ablation. Obstet Gynecol 1999; 94(4):521–7.
38. Vercellini P, Oldani S, DeGiorgi O, et al. Endometrial ablation with a vaporizing electrode in women with regular uterine cavity or submucous leiomyomas. J Am Assoc Gynecol Laparosc 1996;3(4 Suppl):S52.
39. Karandy EJ, Dick HJ, Dwyer RP, et al. Fatal air embolism; a report of two cases, including a case of paradoxical air embolism. Am J Obstet Gynecol 1959;78(1): 96–9.
40. Corson SL, Brooks PG, Soderstrom RM. Gynecologic endoscopic gas embolism. Fertil Steril 1996;65(3):529–33.
41. Perry PM, Baughman VL. A complication of hysteroscopy: air embolism. Anesthesiology 1990;73(3):546–7.
42. Brooks PG. Venous air embolism during operative hysteroscopy. J Am Assoc Gynecol Laparosc 1997;4(3):399–402.
43. Baggish MS, Daniell JF. Death caused by air embolism associated with neodymium: yttrium-aluminum-garnet laser surgery and artificial sapphire tips. Am J Obstet Gynecol 1989;161(4):877–8.
44. Nachum Z, Kol S, Adir Y, et al. Massive air embolism–a possible cause of death after operative hysteroscopy using a 32% dextran-70 pump. Fertil Steril 1992; 58(4):836–8.
45. Groenman FA, Peters LW, Rademaker BM, et al. Embolism of air and gas in hysteroscopic procedures: pathophysiology and implication for daily practice. J Minim Invasive Gynecol 2008;15(2):241–7.

46. Brandner P, Neis KJ, Ehmer C. The etiology, frequency, and prevention of gas embolism during CO_2 hysteroscopy. J Am Assoc Gynecol Laparosc 1999; 6(4):421–8.

47. Obenhaus T, Maurer W. [CO_2 embolism during hysteroscopy]. Anaesthesist 1990;39(4):243–6 [in German].

48. Vo Van JM, Nguyen NQ, Le Bervet JY. [A fatal gas embolism during a hysteroscopy-curettage]. Cah Anesthesiol 1992;40(8):617–8 [in French].

49. Stoloff DR, Isenberg RA, Brill AI. Venous air and gas emboli in operative hysteroscopy. J Am Assoc Gynecol Laparosc 2001;8(2):181–92.

50. Leibowitz D, Benshalom N, Kaganov Y, et al. The incidence and haemodynamic significance of gas emboli during operative hysteroscopy: a prospective echocardiographic study. Eur J Echocardiogr 2010;11(5):429–31.

51. Munro MG, Weisberg M, Rubinstein E. Gas and air embolization during hysteroscopic electrosurgical vaporization: comparison of gas generation using bipolar and monopolar electrodes in an experimental model. J Am Assoc Gynecol Laparosc 2001;8(4):488–94.

52. Munro MG, Brill AI, Ryan T, et al. Electrosurgery-induced generation of gases: comparison of in vitro rates of production using bipolar and monopolar electrodes. J Am Assoc Gynecol Laparosc 2003;10(2):252–9.

53. Karuparthy VR, Downing JW, Husain FJ, et al. Incidence of venous air embolism during cesarean section is unchanged by the use of a 5 to 10 degree head-up tilt. Anesth Analg 1989;69(5):620–3.

54. Handler JS, Bromage PR. Venous air embolism during cesarean delivery. Reg Anesth 1990;15(4):170–3.

55. Durant TM, Long J, Oppenheimer J. Pulmonary venous embolism. Am Heart J 1947;33:269–81.

56. Truhlar A, Cerny V, Dostal P, et al. Out-of-hospital cardiac arrest from air embolism during sexual intercourse: case report and review of the literature. Resuscitation 2007;73(3):475–84.

57. Sullivan B, Kenney P, Seibel M. Hysteroscopic resection of fibroid with thermal injury to sigmoid. Obstet Gynecol 1992;80(3 Pt 2):546–7.

58. Castaing N, Darai E, Chuong T, et al. [Mechanical and metabolic complications of hysteroscopic surgery: report of a retrospective study of 352 procedures]. Contracept Fertil Sex 1999;27(3):210–5 [in French].

59. Agostini A, Cravello L, Desbriere R, et al. Hemorrhage risk during operative hysteroscopy. Acta Obstet Gynecol Scand 2002;81(9):878–81.

60. Munro MG. Mechanisms of thermal injury to the lower genital tract with radiofrequency resectoscopic surgery. J Minim Invasive Gynecol 2006;13(1):36–42.

61. Vilos GA, Brown S, Graham G, et al. Genital tract electrical burns during hysteroscopic endometrial ablation: report of 13 cases in the United States and Canada. J Am Assoc Gynecol Laparosc 2000;7(1):141–7.

62. Vilos GA, Newton DW, Odell RC, et al. Characterization and mitigation of stray radiofrequency currents during monopolar resectoscopic electrosurgery. J Minim Invasive Gynecol 2006;13(2):134–40.

63. Munro MG. Factors affecting capacitive current diversion with a uterine resectoscope: an in vitro study. J Am Assoc Gynecol Laparosc 2003;10(4): 450–60.

64. Chang PT, Vilos GA, Abu-Rafea B, et al. Comparison of clinical outcomes with low-voltage (cut) versus high-voltage (coag) waveforms during hysteroscopic endometrial ablation with the rollerball: a pilot study. J Minim Invasive Gynecol 2009;16(3):350–3.

65. Agostini A, Cravello L, Shojai R, et al. Postoperative infection and surgical hysteroscopy. Fertil Steril 2002;77(4):766–8.
66. McCausland VM, Fields GA, McCausland AM, et al. Tuboovarian abscesses after operative hysteroscopy. J Reprod Med 1993;38(3):198–200.
67. Bhattacharya S, Parkin DE, Reid TM, et al. A prospective randomised study of the effects of prophylactic antibiotics on the incidence of bacteraemia following hysteroscopic surgery. Eur J Obstet Gynecol Reprod Biol 1995;63(1):37–40.
68. Thinkhamrop J, Laopaiboon M, Lumbiganon P. Prophylactic antibiotics for transcervical intrauterine procedures. Cochrane Database Syst Rev 2007;3: CD005637.
69. ACOG Committee on Practice Bulletins-Gynecology. ACOG practice bulletin No. 104: antibiotic prophylaxis for gynecologic procedures. Obstet Gynecol 2009; 113(5):1180–9.
70. Townsend DE, McCausland V, McCausland A, et al. Post-ablation-tubal sterilization syndrome. Obstet Gynecol 1993;82(3):422–4.
71. Sentilhes L, Sergent F, Roman H, et al. Late complications of operative hysteroscopy: predicting patients at risk of uterine rupture during subsequent pregnancy. Eur J Obstet Gynecol Reprod Biol 2005;120(2):134–8.
72. Lo JS, Pickersgill A. Pregnancy after endometrial ablation: English literature review and case report. J Minim Invasive Gynecol 2006;13(2):88–91.
73. Patni S, ElGarib AM, Majd HS, et al. Endometrial resection mandates reliable contraception thereafter - a case report of placenta increta following endometrial ablation. Eur J Contracept Reprod Health Care 2008;13(2):208–11.
74. Laberge PY. Serious and deadly complications from pregnancy after endometrial ablation: two case reports and review of the literature. J Gynecol Obstet Biol Reprod (Paris) 2008;37(6):609–13.

Gynecologic Surgery and the Management of Hemorrhage

William H. Parker, MD[a],*, Willis H. Wagner, MD[b]

KEYWORDS

- Gynecologic surgery • Hemorrhage • Hemostasis

Surgical blood loss of more than 1000 mL or blood loss that requires a blood transfusion usually defines intraoperative hemorrhage.[1] Intraoperative hemorrhage has been reported in 1% to 2% of hysterectomy studies.

Acute loss of more than 25% of the patient's blood volume or a loss that is sufficient to require an intervention to save the patient's life defines massive hemorrhage.[2] Cardiovascular instability with significant hypotension often results from a loss of 30% to 40% of the patient's blood volume. More than 40% blood loss is life threatening. Severe hemorrhage can lead to multiorgan failure and death unless resuscitation is accomplished within an hour.

Severe postoperative anemia can affect mortality. In a study of 300 patients who refused blood transfusion for religious reasons, it was found that patients with hemoglobin levels of 5.1 to 7.0 g/dL had mortality of 9%. Mortality was 30% in patients with hemoglobin levels between 3.1 and 5.0 g/dL and 64% in those with hemoglobin levels less than 3.0 g/dL. However, hemoglobin levels between 7 and 8 g/dL did not have any adverse effect on mortality.[3]

PREOPERATIVE EVALUATION

Preoperative evaluation of the patient can aid surgical planning to help prevent intraoperative hemorrhage or prepare for the management of hemorrhage, should it occur.

Medical History

Personal or family history of prolonged bleeding, postpartum hemorrhage, need for transfusions, or persistent anemia should be determined. von Willebrand disease (VWD) occurs in 2% of women in the general population; however, 17% of women

[a] Department of Obstetrics and Gynecology, Saint John's Health Center, University of California Los Angeles School of Medicine, 1450 Tenth Street, Santa Monica, Los Angeles, CA 90401, USA
[b] Vascular Laboratory, Saint John's Health Center, 2121 Santa Monica Boulevard, Santa Monica, CA 90404, USA
* Corresponding author.
E-mail address: wparker@ucla.edu

Obstet Gynecol Clin N Am 37 (2010) 427–436
doi:10.1016/j.ogc.2010.05.003
0889-8545/10/$ – see front matter © 2010 Elsevier Inc. All rights reserved.

obgyn.theclinics.com

with menorrhagia have VWD. Because menorrhagia is a common indication for gynecologic surgery, a history of menorrhagia since menarche should trigger further evaluation by a hematologist. If the diagnosis is made, desmopressin (DDAVP) can be used to reduce intraoperative bleeding by increasing the plasma concentration and activity of von Willebrand factor. Women with religious beliefs that preclude transfusion with allogenic blood should be identified before elective surgery. Increasing hemoglobin concentrations before surgery should be strongly considered (see later sections).

Medication History

Because coagulation may be inhibited by medications, including prescription, over-the-counter, or alternative formulations, the surgeon should inquire about the use of these substances. Patients often do not mention these products.

Aspirin, often used for fever, headache, or pain should be discontinued 7 to 10 days before surgery. Aspirin inhibits platelet cyclooxygenase within 1 hour of ingestion.[4] This effect is irreversible, so platelet aggregation studies can give abnormal results for up to 10 days. Nonsteroidal antiinflammatory drugs (NSAIDs) cause inhibition of cyclooxygenase, which is reversible. Platelet function returns to normal within 24 hours after the last dose of ibuprofen, but with most other NSAIDs platelet function is abnormal for 3 days.[5]

Clopidogrel bisulfate (Plavix), a long-acting oral antiplatelet medication, causes a dose-dependent inhibition of platelet aggregation 2 hours after the first dose. With continued use, it takes about 5 days after treatment is discontinued for bleeding time to return to normal. A 1.5% increase in the frequency of surgical bleeding events was reported in a meta-analysis of men and women taking low-dose aspirin and undergoing noncardiac surgeries and invasive procedures. However, neither the severity of bleeding complications nor the perioperative mortality increased for abdominal surgery.[6]

Patients with a history of cardiovascular disease or thrombosis who take aspirin or Plavix for prophylaxis should be managed jointly with an internist. Continued use of these drugs depends on the potential risk of thrombotic complications that arise if aspirin is discontinued versus the risks of perioperative bleeding associated with continued therapy.[7] Stopping aspirin therapy for more than 5 days in patients with underlying cardiovascular disease may increase the risk of an acute coronary syndrome or stroke. Management of warfarin or heparin should also be coordinated by the prescribing clinician.

Alternative Medications

Impaired hemostasis has been shown to be more than 2 times as likely for patients using traditional Chinese herbal medicines than for nonusers.[8] Garlic, Ginkgo biloba, and ginseng may also affect coagulation through the inhibition of platelet aggregation.[9]

Preoperative Laboratory Evaluation

- A baseline hematocrit (Hct) should be obtained before surgery, preferably in time to allow for correction of anemia, if found. In the gynecologic population, the most common form of anemia is iron deficiency anemia caused by menorrhagia or dietary deficiency.
- Blood typing and antibody screening should be performed for patients undergoing surgery with expected blood loss. Typing and crossmatching of 2 to 4 units

of packed red blood cells (RBCs) (and/or the use of a cell saver, see later section) should be considered if significant bleeding is anticipated.

- Routine tests of hemostasis (prothrombin time [PT], activated partial thromboplastin time [aPTT], and platelet count) are not necessary unless the patient has a known bleeding diathesis, an illness that is associated with bleeding tendency, or has used medication that has the potential to cause anticoagulation. If VWD is suspected, evaluation by an internist or hematologist is helpful. If VWD is detected, treatment with DDAVP just before surgery can reverse the clotting defect.

PREOPERATIVE MANAGEMENT OF ANEMIA
Iron Therapy

If possible, iron deficiency anemia should be treated before surgery with elemental iron, 150 to 200 mg/d. Iron should not be taken with food because food binds with iron and decreases its absorption. However, taking vitamin C, 250 mg, with iron enhances the iron absorption. Side effects include nausea, constipation, or epigastric distress for about 10% to 20% of patients taking oral iron. The hemoglobin concentration increases slowly, usually beginning after about 1 to 2 weeks of treatment, and increases by approximately 2 g/dL during the ensuing 3 weeks. In the absence of continued bleeding, the hemoglobin level should return to normal by 6 to 8 weeks.

Recombinant Erythropoietin

Although not often considered by gynecologists, recombinant forms of erythropoietin (Epo) are commonly used to increase preoperative hemoglobin concentrations in cardiac, orthopedic, and neurologic surgeries. To be effective, iron stores must be adequate and iron should be given before or concurrently with Epo. When significant blood loss is anticipated in women who will not accept blood products, Epo may be used to increase the hemoglobin concentration preoperatively.

A randomized study showed that the use of Epo, approximately 15,000 U/wk, for 3 weeks before elective surgery increased the hemoglobin concentration by 1.6 g/dL. A significant reduction in the need for transfusions was noted when compared with controls.[10] A prospective, nonrandomized study of gynecologic surgery found a significant increase in hemoglobin concentrations after preoperative use of epoetin.[11] Epo has been associated with cardiovascular and thrombotic events in patients with cancer who used the drug repetitively during chemotherapy. However, these problems have not been reported for short-term use in healthy women.

Gonadotropin-Releasing Hormone Agonists

Gonadotropin-releasing hormone agonists (GnRH-as) may be used preoperatively to stop abnormal uterine bleeding and increase hemoglobin concentrations. Women scheduled for surgery for fibroid-related problems who had mean hemoglobin concentrations of 10.2 g/dL were randomized preoperatively to a combination of GnRH-a and oral iron or placebo and oral iron. After 12 weeks, 74% of the women treated with GnRH-a and iron had hemoglobin levels greater than 12 g/dL compared with 46% of the women treated with iron alone.[12] Side effects, including hot flashes, insomnia, vaginal dryness, and headaches, may limit the use of GnRH-a.

Autologous Blood Donation

Autologous blood donation has a decreased risk of human immunodeficiency virus (HIV) or hepatitis infection and hemolytic, febrile, or allergic transfusion reactions. However, this concept assumes that no clerical errors result in the inadvertent transfusion of the wrong unit of blood. Autologous units should be drawn weekly, with the last unit drawn 2 weeks before surgery.

INTRAOPERATIVE MANAGEMENT OF HEMORRHAGE
Initial Interventions

The initial step to control hemorrhage is tamponade. Pressure should be applied with fingers or a sponge stick to the bleeding area, allowing the patient to be stabilized while other measures are taken. During laparotomy, if localized pressure does not control bleeding, damp laparotomy pads may be firmly placed against the bleeding site. Pressure needs to be applied for 10 to 15 minutes, and the packs should be observed to confirm that bleeding has stopped.

During laparoscopic surgery, an atraumatic laparoscopic grasper may be applied to the site of small-vessel bleeding. If large vessel bleeding occurs because of trocar injury, one or two 4 × 8 inch gauze sponges may be pushed through the 10-mm umbilical port and pressure applied to the bleeding area. It is not likely that this type of injury can be repaired laparoscopically; therefore, a vertical midline incision should be made, and tamponade can then be applied with "laparotomy" sponges. A vertical incision allows the vascular surgeon access to the aorta, vena cava, and iliac vessels, which are the most common areas of injury.

Whereas securing hemostasis is critical, care should be taken to avoid tissue necrosis, organ injury, vascular thrombosis, fistula formation, or nerve dysfunction.[13] Once the bleeding area is identified and tamponade applied, identifying the ureter and major vessels can help to avoid injuries to these structures.

The anesthesia team should be informed of the potential for significant blood loss. The patient's hemodynamic status should be immediately assessed by the anesthesiologist and communicated to the surgeon, and the dialogue should continue until the situation is under control. Fluid replacement for hemorrhage should be given in crystalloid fluid/blood loss ratio of 3:1. Additional monitoring and the ordering of blood replacement products should be considered if indicated. The surgeon, anesthesiologist, and operating room team should discuss and coordinate the next steps. A moment of calm and time for organization allows clearer thinking and avoids actions based on panic and fear, which are not likely to be productive and may, in fact, do harm. Often, the continued application of pressure while waiting for a vascular or general surgeon may be the best course of action. Injudicious attempts at obtaining vascular control may worsen the injury, particularly in major retroperitoneal veins.

The need for assistance should be discussed, including another anesthesiologist to assist with placement of arterial and central venous lines, additional nursing support, additional help to transport laboratory and blood products and, if necessary, an additional surgeon with expertise in vascular surgery.

If the blood bank does not have a current blood sample, a sample should be sent to be typed and crossmatched. Hct, platelet count, PT level, and aPTT should be checked. (See section on blood transfusion). Frequent communication between members of the operating room team and blood bank regarding patient status and the need for blood products should continue until hemostasis is certain.

Intraoperative Blood Salvage with Cell Savers

Cell savers have been used extensively in orthopedic, cardiac, and neurologic surgeries and should be considered for use during gynecologic surgery when bleeding is anticipated or occurs. The device suctions blood from the operative field, mixes it with heparinized saline, and stores the blood in a canister. If the patient requires blood reinfusion, the stored blood is washed with saline, filtered, centrifuged to an Hct of approximately 50%, and given back to the patient in the operating room.[14] When rapid bleeding is encountered, the cell saver can provide the equivalent of 12 units of banked blood per hour. Although the posttransfusion survival of the red cells is excellent, cell-saver blood lacks functional platelets, white cells, and coagulation factors. Use of the cell saver avoids the risks of infection and transfusion reaction. Also, cell-saver blood may be accepted by some women who do not accept transfusion for religious reasons.

Identifying the Source of Bleeding

Bleeding from the intravenous insertion site and all operative sites indicates possible disseminated intravascular coagulation and should be treated medically. The following are the most common sites of major blood loss in the pelvis (cephalad to caudad): inferior vena cava, presacral veins, ovarian vessels, common and external iliac vessels, internal iliac vessels, parametrial and paracervical varicosities, and the bladder pillars and posterior bladder. The vascular structures of the reproductive tract are confined within the tissues that separate the avascular spaces—the paravesical, pararectal, vesicovaginal, and rectovaginal spaces. Development of the appropriate space often allows control of bleeding sites while avoiding trauma to important pelvic structures.[13]

The pararectal space is bounded by the internal iliac artery laterally and the ureter medially and can be approached by incision of the pelvic peritoneum (and preferably the round ligament) lateral to the iliac vessels. Separation of the vessels and the ureter and a posterior and slightly medial dissection exposes the proximal pelvic ureter, the internal iliac vessels, and the rectum. The paravesical space is bounded by the external iliac vessels laterally and the obliterated hypogastric artery (medial umbilical ligament) medially, and dissection of this space exposes the lateral portions of the bladder, vagina, and rectum.

The walls of the major veins are delicate; so care should be taken during dissection to avoid injury and brisk bleeding. Small tributaries from the common iliac vein, inferior vena cava, pelvic sidewall, or the presacral veins can avulse during blunt dissection, with resultant high-volume bleeding.

Control of Bleeding

Electrosurgery, suture, or surgical clips can be used to control small-vessel bleeding. Vessels should be isolated, and vital structures identified before ligation is performed to avoid inadvertent injury. Mass suture or indiscriminate use of electrosurgery or clips should be avoided. For small-vessel injury and oozing, consideration should be given to packing followed by arterial embolization if bleeding continues. It should be noted that ligation of the internal iliac artery (discussed later in the section on internal iliac artery ligation) precludes subsequent embolization.

The most difficult type of bleeding to control, venous bleeding, reflects the high volume of blood flowing through fragile, irregular veins. Gentle pressure with sponge sticks on either side of the venous injury is the most useful method to control and minimize blood loss. Usually, it is better to avoid pressure packing, which may increase the risk of venous stasis and pelvic or distal venous thrombosis. The placement of hemoclips often controls bleeding. However, application of hemoclips to a peg hole defect in a way that reduces the caliber of the lumen may lead to thrombosis.

A vascular surgeon should be called to repair the aorta, vena cava, and common and external iliac vessels, which perfuse the extremities. In general, these vessels are repaired by compressing the vessel above and below the injury with vascular clamps and suturing the defect with a running 4-0 to 6-0 monofilament suture with a cardiovascular needle. In a nonirradiated pelvis, the extensive arterial collateral circulation in the peripheral pelvis allows ligation of internal iliac vessels.[13]

The venous plexus over the presacral area may be a particularly difficult area to control bleeding. Although pressure, electrosurgery, clips, or sutures may work, pressing a sterile steel thumbtack directly into the bone at the bleeding site may be more effective.

Internal iliac artery ligation

If initial attempts to achieve hemostasis are not successful, the next step is to decrease pelvic blood flow. Bilateral internal iliac artery ligation lowers the rate of blood flow to the pelvis by half and lowers the pulse pressure of the vasculature by 85%. Therefore, ligation reduces the arterial pressure to form a low-pressure system, which is more amenable to clot formation.

If necessary, internal iliac ligation is performed by initially opening the retroperitoneal space laterally and parallel to the ureters and retracting the peritoneum and ureter medially. The internal iliac artery is then dissected until the posterior branch is identified. A right-angled clamp is placed distal to the posterior branch, taking care not to injure the iliac vein below. Two ligatures are placed around the internal iliac vessel at this point to secure it. The external iliac artery should be palpated to confirm that its blood supply has not been compromised. The procedure should then be repeated on the opposite side.[15] Ligation of the internal iliac artery should only be performed by surgeons who are experienced with this procedure.

Topical hemostatic agents

Topical hemostatic agents are effective for control of diffuse, low-volume venous bleeding sites. There are no controlled studies that compare topical hemostatic agents with each other or with alternate means of controlling bleeding.

- Gelfoam/thrombin (Pfizer, Inc, New York, NY, USA), an absorbable gelatin matrix, can be cut into any shape to facilitate application. Gelfoam is rigid when dry, but when thrombin is applied to Gelfoam it becomes more pliable and may be passed through laparoscopic trocars. Thrombin makes the Gelfoam patch hemostatic; pressure should be applied to the patch for several minutes, and then the patch is left in place. These items are generally available in most operating rooms and are probably the most cost-effective agents for hemostasis.
- Surgicel (Ethicon, New Brunswick, NJ, USA), made of oxidized regenerated cellulose, can be applied dry, directly to the bleeding areas. Also, Surgicel is pliable and can be rolled and passed easily through laparoscopic trocars. Excessive use of Surgicel may cause infection, fibrosis, or adhesions.
- FloSeal (Baxter, Deerfield, IL, USA) is a hemostatic agent that may be used in situations in which diffuse oozing is present. The solution is made from human plasma and constituted by mixing gelatin and thrombin. The solution may then be directly applied to bleeding sites.
- Tisseel (Baxter, Deerfield, IL, USA) may also be used when diffuse bleeding is present. This product is a mixture of thrombin and highly concentrated human fibrinogen and can be directly sprayed onto bleeding sites.

Pelvic packing

If other measures do not control bleeding in the pelvis, a pressure pack may be left in the pelvis for 48 to 72 hours. A sterile plastic radiograph film cover is filled with rolls of gauze knotted together, the tail of the gauze is left protruding through the bag's opening, and the drawstrings are tightened. Taking care to avoid bowel or ovary entrapment, the pack is placed into the pelvis and the drawstrings and gauze tail are pulled through the vaginal cuff.[15]

To maintain constant pressure, a 1000 mL intravenous fluid bag is attached to the pack with surgical tubing and hung off the end of the bed. A Jackson-Pratt drain is also placed in the pelvis so that continued bleeding can be monitored. An indwelling urinary catheter avoids outflow obstruction by the pack and allows urine output to be monitored. After 48 to 72 hours, with decreasing vaginal and Jackson-Pratt drain output, the gauze can be slowly removed from the pack over 4 hours. The bag can then be removed through the vagina and the vaginal cuff left open for any further drainage.[16]

Significant intraperitoneal or retroperitoneal bleeding can lead to increased intra-abdominal pressure and abdominal compartment syndrome. The increased intra-abdominal pressure can be transmitted to the pleural space, causing a decrease in lung compliance and hypoxemia and a decrease in venous return. Decreased perfusion of the intra-abdominal organs can lead to oliguria and renal failure.[17]

Mast suits, which further increase intra-abdominal pressure, are not indicated for controlling ongoing intra-abdominal bleeding.

POSTOPERATIVE BLEEDING

Mobilization of fluids postoperatively can lead to a drop in hemoglobin level without any ongoing bleeding. After hysterectomy, ongoing vaginal bleeding is often the first sign of bleeding. Tachycardia, hypotension, distension, oliguria, confusion, sweating, and increasing abdominal pain may all signal intra-abdominal bleeding after surgery. If the bleeding is minimal, observation with serial hemoglobin measurements and transfusion may be considered, but the need for repeated transfusion should trigger a more aggressive response.

Careful monitoring of blood pressure, urine output, and central venous pressure can help in diagnosing ongoing bleeding. If the patient's condition deteriorates in the absence of obvious bleeding, then retroperitoneal bleeding should be considered. If the patient is stable, a computed tomographic scan can be helpful in evaluating the amount of blood in the retroperitoneal space or free in the abdomen. Small retroperitoneal hematomas may tamponade and then eventually be reabsorbed. Patients with shock and increasing abdominal girth should be surgically reexplored immediately.

Embolization

Embolization can be used to occlude the vessels feeding the pelvis. The procedure may take up to 2 hours and can be considered for women with active arterial bleeding but who are otherwise hemodynamically stable. Preoperative embolization has been used for procedures in which the risk of hemorrhage is thought to be high.

Endografts

Patients with postoperative bleeding caused by injury to the vena cava or common or external iliac veins can be successfully treated with stented grafts that are inserted by an endovascular specialist under radiologic guidance.

TRANSFUSIONS

Guidelines for red cell transfusions and volume replacement in adults are based on the estimation of blood loss.[18] Patient concerns about infection (HIV or hepatitis) should be discussed in the light of the markedly decreased incidence currently reported by most blood banks: HIV, 1 infected unit per 2 million units transfused; hepatitis B, 1 unit per 200,000 units transfused; and hepatitis C, 1 unit per 2 million units transfused.

Blood Loss Less Than 750 mL

These patients do not require transfusion unless they have preexisting anemia or are unable to compensate because of severe cardiac or respiratory disease.

Blood Loss from 800 to 1500 mL

RBC transfusion is usually unnecessary unless the patient has preexisting anemia, continuing blood loss, or reduced cardiovascular reserve.

Blood Loss from 1500 to 2000 mL

These patients require rapid volume replacement with crystalloids or synthetic colloids and probably RBC transfusion.

Blood Loss of More Than 2000 mL

These patients require rapid volume replacement including RBC transfusion.

Each unit of packed cells contains approximately 200 mL of red cells. In an adult with no further bleeding, 1 unit of blood increases the Hct by 3% to 4% points and the hemoglobin by 1 g/dL. The PT, aPTT, and platelet count should be frequently monitored, preferably after each 5 units of blood replaced. If the PT and aPTT exceed 1.5 times the control value, the patient should be transfused with 2 units of fresh frozen plasma. If the platelet count decreases to less than 50,000/mL, 6 units of platelets should be given.

Acid-base balance and plasma calcium and potassium levels should be checked periodically, especially in patients with liver or renal disease. Acidosis does not usually develop if tissue perfusion is maintained. Citrate, used to anticoagulate stored blood, binds to calcium and can cause a decrease in plasma calcium levels. The level of plasma potassium increases in stored blood, but even a significant transfusion usually does not lead to an increase in the plasma potassium level, except in patients with renal impairment.

AVOIDING COAGULOPATHY

A systolic blood pressure less than 70 mm Hg, acidosis (pH <7.1), and hypothermia (temperature <34°C) inhibit clotting enzymes and increase the risk of coagulopathy.[19] Infusion of large volumes of crystalloid and colloidal fluids and transfusion of packed RBCs dilute the clotting factors and platelets, also predisposing the patient to coagulopathy.[20]

There are no universally accepted guidelines for blood component therapy. Replacement of RBCs, platelets, plasma, and fibrinogen or cryoprecipitate is best used according to the patient's needs.[21] Component therapy is used when there is clinical evidence of coagulopathy, microvascular diffuse bleeding, or abnormal results in laboratory tests. Blood component treatment should be considered when a patient has microvascular bleeding, an Hct less than 24%, a PT or aPTT more than 1.5 times the normal, a platelet count less than 50,000/mL, or a fibrinogen concentration less than 1 g/L. Patients who are taking Plavix or have recently taken aspirin are likely to have platelet dysfunction even in the presence of a normal platelet count, and these patients should be considered for early administration of platelets.

Some investigators suggest empiric administration of blood products[22]:

- Perform primary volume expansion before replacing blood or blood components.
- For every 8 U of RBCs transfused, give 2 U of fresh frozen plasma.
- If more than 10 U of RBCs are replaced, give 10 U of platelets, preferably at the end of the procedure. With prolonged aPTT, give fresh frozen plasma.
- If fibrinogen is low, give 2 U of cryoprecipitate. One option when facing massive hemorrhage is to give cryoprecipitate initially.

Often, early involvement of a hematologist is of help when managing patients with massive bleeding or a coagulopathy.

REFERENCES

1. Harris WJ. Early complications of abdominal and vaginal hysterectomy. Obstet Gynecol Surv 1995;50:795–805.
2. Santoso JT, Saunders BA, Grosshart K. Massive blood loss and transfusion in obstetrics and gynecology. Obstet Gynecol Surv 2005;60:827–37.
3. Carson JL, Noveck H, Berlin JA, et al. Mortality and morbidity in patients with very low postoperative Hb levels who decline blood transfusion. Transfusion 2002;42:812.
4. Patrono C, Ciabattoni G, Pinca E, et al. Low dose aspirin and inhibition of thromboxane B2 production in healthy subjects. Thromb Res 1980;17:317.
5. Goldenberg NA, Jacobson L, Manco-Johnson MJ. Brief communication: duration of platelet dysfunction after a 7-day course of ibuprofen. Ann Intern Med 2005; 142:506.
6. Burger W, Chemnitius JM, Kneissl GD, et al. Low dose aspirin for secondary cardiovascular prevention—cardiovascular risks after its perioperative withdrawal versus bleeding risks with its continuation—review and meta-analysis. J Intern Med 2005;257:399.
7. Kroenke K, Goobey-Toedt D, Jacksno JL. Chronic medications in the perioperative period. South Med J 1998;91:358.
8. Lee A, Chui PT, Aun CS, et al. Incidence and risk of adverse perioperative events among surgical patients taking traditional Chinese herbal medicines. Anesthesiology 2006;105:454.
9. Ang-Lee MK, Moss J, Yuan CS. Herbal medicines and perioperative care. JAMA 2001;286:208.
10. Wurnig C, Schatz K, Noske H, et al. Subcutaneous low-dose epoetin beta for the avoidance of transfusion in patients scheduled for elective surgery not eligible for autologous blood donation. Eur Surg Res 2001;33:303–10.
11. Sesti F, Ticconi C, Bonifacio S, et al. Preoperative administration of recombinant human erythropoietin in patients undergoing gynecologic surgery. Gynecol Obstet Invest 2002;54:1–5.
12. de Aloysio D, Altieri P, Pretolani G, et al. The combined effect of a GnRH analog in premenopause plus postmenopausal estrogen deficiency for the treatment of uterine leiomyomas in perimenopausal women. Gynecol Obstet Invest 1995;39:115–9.
13. Gostout B, Cliby W, Podratz C. Prevention and management of acute intraoperative bleeding. Clin Obstet Gynecol 2002;45:481–91.
14. West S, Ruiz R, Parker WH. Abdominal myomectomy in women with very large uterine size. Fertil Steril 2006;85:36–9.
15. Tamizian O, Arulkumaran S. The surgical management of postpartum haemorrhage. Curr Opin Obstet Gynecol 2001;13:127–31.

16. Howard R, Straughn M, Huh W, et al. Pelvic umbrella pack for refractory obstetric hemorrhage secondary to posterior uterine rupture. Obstet Gynecol 2002;100: 1061–3.

17. Balogh Z, Jones F, D'Amours S, et al. Continuous intra-abdominal pressure measurement technique. Am J Surg 2004;188:679–84.

18. Murphy MF, Wallington TB, Kelsey P, et al. British committee for standards in haematology, blood transfusion task force. Br J Haematol 2001;113:24–31.

19. Cosgriff N, Moore EE, Sauia A, et al. Predicting life-threatening coagulopathy in the massively transfused trauma patient. Hypothermia and acidosis revisited. J Trauma 1997;42:857–61.

20. Hardy JF, Samama M. Massive transfusion and coagulopathy. Transfus Altern Transfus Med 2003;4:199–210.

21. Erber WN. Massive blood transfusion in the elective surgery setting. Transfus Apheresis Sci 2002;27:83–92.

22. Hiippala S. Replacement of massive blood loss. Vox Sang 1998;74(Suppl 2): 399–407.

Understanding Errors During Laparoscopic Surgery

William H. Parker, MD

KEYWORDS

- Laparoscopic complications • Surgical error
- Surgery and cognitive science
- Surgery and crew resource management

Complications may occur during laparoscopic surgery, even with a skilled, experienced surgeon and under ideal circumstances. Human error is inevitable.

An understanding of the limitations of the human brain may help surgeons navigate through difficult surgical situations and, perhaps, even avoid complications.[1] Problems with visual perception and processing, loss of haptic perception, poor performance under stress, and lack of situation awareness may lead to surgical complications.[2] Long-term memory is also critical to the successful performance of surgery; semantic memory (book-learned anatomy, instrument function), procedural memory (how to perform a procedure), and episodic memory (an individual's past experiences during surgery) are important components.

The role that the human brain's hardwiring (connections among neurons) plays in shaping information processing and the role that perceptual learning and situation awareness play during the performance of surgical procedures are considered here. Surgical error prevention and management and the structure of surgical training are also discussed. The following case presentations are derived from real videotaped procedures in which malpractice was alleged, and these cases were resolved in court.

VISUAL ERRORS
Surgical Video: Case 1

A 25-year-old woman is undergoing a diagnostic laparoscopy to determine the cause of her chronic pelvic pain. The initial view of the pelvis clearly shows normal anatomy without evidence of adhesions, endometriosis, or other pathologic conditions. The surgeon decides to perform a laparoscopic uterosacral nerve ablation to treat her pelvic pain.

Department of Obstetrics and Gynecology, Saint John's Health Center, University of California Los Angeles School of Medicine, 1450 Tenth Street, Santa Monica, Los Angeles, CA 90401, USA
E-mail address: wparker@ucla.edu

Obstet Gynecol Clin N Am 37 (2010) 437–449
doi:10.1016/j.ogc.2010.06.001
0889-8545/10/$ – see front matter © 2010 Elsevier Inc. All rights reserved.

obgyn.theclinics.com

We see an Nd:YAG laser fiber passed down the operating channel of the laparoscope and directed toward a prominent structure on the right pelvic sidewall, near the cul-de-sac. The laparoscope is moved close to the structure, narrowing the field of view, and the YAG fiber contacts the tissue. The laser is activated, and the structure is severed. The surgeon's attention is turned to the mirror-image structure on the left pelvic sidewall, which is also severed. The laparoscope is pulled back, both ovaries are deflected to show a panoramic view of the pelvis, and the procedure is terminated. The panoramic view clearly shows that both ureters have been transected lateral to the uterosacral ligaments.

However, the injury is not appreciated, and the patient is discharged. She returns the following day with acute abdominal pain, nausea, and vomiting. At laparotomy, the abdomen is filled with urine, and reimplantation of both ureters is required.

The cognitive principle of tunnel vision is demonstrated in **Fig. 1**. Although initially it may be difficult to pick out the Dalmatian, once the brain constructs the dog out of the various shapes it is almost impossible to make the image go away. The brain tries to organize incoming sensations into information that is meaningful and holds on to those images. Surgical case 1 illustrates the same cognitive process. In this video, once a quick determination was made about the identity of the uterosacral ligament, the imprint was preserved by the brain. When the brain forms these quick impressions, it excludes other contradictory information, and it is hard to redirect the cognitive process to include more information.

In **Fig. 2**, a larger triangle surrounding a smaller one is likely to be seen. However, the figure consists of only 6 Pacman-like shapes. When encountered in the real world, these patterns are most likely to come from triangles, so the brain constructs shapes that are expected, causing an optical illusion. Usually these perceptual principles work pretty well, but not always as demonstrated by surgical case 1.

The human mind is an incredible achievement, but not perfectly designed. The neural connections of the human brain are designed to quickly learn patterns in the environment. Of the 11,000,000 bits of perceptual information entering the brain every second, only 40 are consciously processed.[3] Because of this limitation, the brain tries to chunk things together when it needs to manage complexity.[4] To do this, our

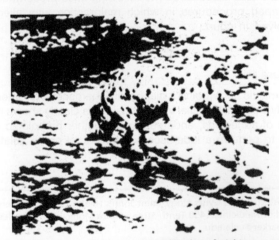

Fig. 1. Dalmatian dog. This picture illustrates the difficulty of picking out the meaning from a sparse or noisy image. But once seen in a certain way, the brain holds on to that image. *From* Gregory R. The intelligent eye. McGraw-Hill Book Company; 1970.

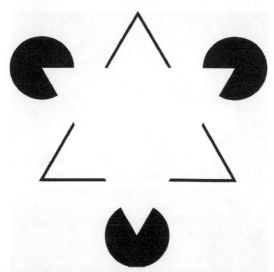

Fig. 2. Some circles, some lines, but no white triangle. (*From* http://commons.wikimedia.org/wiki/File:Kanizsa_triangle.svg. Accessed July 7, 2010. This figure is licensed under the Creative Commons Attribution-ShareAlike 3.0; with permission.)

unconscious brains quickly construct what is familiar and expected and signal whether these patterns are good or bad.

Rapid, unconscious processing has evolutionary advantages. Early human ancestors who were most skilled at quickly processing information, for example, recognizing a snake in the forest, had a survival advantage. Those who reacted slowly, or mistook the snake for a stick, did not survive to bestow genes to the next generation. But these chunks or shortcuts are inflexible and sometimes error prone.[5]

In surgical case 1, the most prominent and easily seen structures, usually the uterosacral ligaments, were instead the ureters. Both ureters were severed despite visual cues to the contrary; the video clearly shows uterosacral ligaments well below the ureter, and peristalsis can be seen as the ureter is exposed to heat from the laser. Conscious processing, that is, a more detailed analysis of information and environmental cues at the cortical level, is slower but can be more accurate. Being retroperitoneal structures, the ureters can be difficult to see, especially late in the procedure when peritoneal irritation and edema can impair visualization. Identifying the ureters early in the procedure, when they look similar to textbook images, and making small incisions in the peritoneum above the ureters marks them for easy identification later and may help avoid injury (**Fig. 3**).

Laparoscopic surgery has several recognized advantages over abdominal surgery. The laparoscope illuminates and magnifies, effectively allowing the surgeon's eye to get extremely close to the tissue, providing the surgeon with the anatomic detail that is never seen during laparotomy. However, this level of detail comes at a cost. Closely positioning the laparoscope for greater precision precludes a panoramic view of other structures near the operating field. Conversely, a distant wide-angle view allows an overview of other anatomic structures but does not demonstrate the detail necessary for safe manipulation of the instruments and surgical precision (see **Fig. 3**).

The experienced laparoscopic surgeon, usually without conscious awareness, intermittently repositions the laparoscope, changing perspective from close to wide

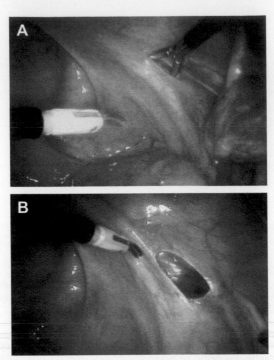

Fig. 3. (*A, B*) Marking ureters. (*From* Parker WH, Johns A, Hellige J. Avoiding complications of laparoscopic surgery: lessons from cognitive science and crew resource management. J Minim Invasive Gynecol 2007;14(3):381; with permission.)

angle and back again and also from right to left. In this way, nearby structures, both those at risk and safe areas, are continually processed and tunnel vision can be avoided. This behavior is akin to an experienced driver glancing, unconsciously, between the road ahead and the side and rear view mirrors. For surgeons in the early and deliberate phases of learning, movement of the laparoscope between near and wide-angle views should be consciously undertaken until these actions become instinctual. At first, the intentional method is slower but reliable. Over time, this processing becomes instinctual and quick. In surgical video 1, even after damage had been done to the first ureter, pulling back the laparoscope to change the view and purposefully reassess the anatomy would have prevented damage to the contralateral ureter.

Similar perceptual/visual problems were documented in a review of 22 unedited videotapes of laparoscopic cholecystectomy procedures ending in litigation.[1] Most often, the common duct was misperceived as the cystic duct and cut. Reviewers found that 97% of the surgeons showed evidence of visual/perception errors, whereas only 3% exhibited evidence of lack of technical skill or knowledge.

ERRORS OF INEXPERIENCE
Surgical Video: Case 2

A 23-year-old woman with chronic pelvic pain and infertility is admitted for a diagnostic laparoscopy. A small area of endometriosis is seen in the posterior cul-de-sac, within a small peritoneal window. The tissue is grasped and elevated, and a carbon-dioxide laser is used to excise it. The tissue is pliable and thick, and a large area is removed.

Review of the video shows the rectum being tented up by the grasper. The laser cuts far under the peritoneum, and stool can be clearly seen oozing out of the injured rectum, unrecognized by the surgeon.

The patient is sent home but returns to the emergency room the next day with fever, vomiting, and signs of an acute abdomen. Emergency laparotomy reveals fecal contents in the abdomen and a 2-cm defect in the anterior rectal wall. A diverting colostomy is performed, and the patient requires readmission months later for laparotomy and bowel reanastomosis. Future fertility has been compromised.

In 1983, an art dealer contacted the J. Paul Getty Museum in Los Angeles about a recently discovered Greek sculpture of a man created in approximately 500 BC.[6] The museum was interested in acquiring the Kouros and took the sculpture on consignment for examination and analysis of its authenticity. For 14 months they evaluated the statue and, convinced of its authenticity, bought the sculpture for US $10 million.

Shortly thereafter, Thomas Hoving, former curator of the Metropolitan Museum of Art in New York, was invited to view the new acquisition. The moment Hoving entered the room, he turned to his colleague and said, "I hope you haven't paid for this yet." Based on this startling first impression, the museum reevaluated the evidence of the statue's authenticity. Document forgery, errors in the dating analysis, and a similarity to a previously known forgery were discovered. Today the statue stands in the museum with the plaque "Kouros, 500 BC, or modern forgery."

How did Hoving see something that 14 months of analysis had not uncovered? The answer is experience. Hoving, an expert in ancient art, had examined thousands of works of art during his 20-year career and had made a habit of noting the first word that came to his mind when he saw a new piece of art. On seeing the Kouros, the first word that instinctively occurred to him was "fresh," an unlikely impression of a statue buried in the ground for more than 2500 years.

Cognitive science describes 2 basic types of thinking: deliberate (knowledge-based) and instinctive (unconscious processing). Deliberate thinking is processed consciously by the cortex, with careful weighing of the pros and cons before a decision is made. Instinctive thinking results from quick decisions processed in the unconscious mind (anterior cingulated gyrus), based on instantly recognized patterns stored in long-term memory. Think about learning to drive a car. In the beginning, driving requires careful attention to the road, the pedals, and other cars and road obstacles. However, with practice, processing all this information becomes essentially automatic. Think about the degree of attention paid to these driving details when listening to a favorite song on the car radio.

With experience and practice, some knowledge-based cognitive behaviors can be relegated to unconscious cognition.[7] Every exposure to the same or similar thing reinforces neural connections and increases the chance that an event makes it into long-term memory, and it is more likely that the response will be accurate. The greater the proficiency the lesser the detailed analysis necessary, and the more that pattern recognition and shortcuts are used the less the energy requirements of the brain. Also, practice, experience, and repeated use of specific memories increase connections between neurons and increase brain areas allocated to a particular skill.[8] Encoding into long-term memory can take years.[9]

The definition of expertise is knowing what to do, rapidly and efficiently.[10] Experts use the conscious mind to acquire as much information as possible. Experts are also careful to study their mistakes, allowing the brain to revise the models it holds in long-term memory. The unconscious mind's neurons are able to process all of this information in parallel, with resulting massive computational power.[4] For chess experts, unconscious processing has been calculated to be equivalent to 125 million bits per second in computer raw search. This degree of processing allows experts to notice details and relationships to which the novice is oblivious, explaining the magical levels of expertise that develop after years of experience in science, chess, mathematics, and music.

Returning to surgical video 2, the area incised was near the rectovaginal septum, so named because of its proximity to the rectum. Clearly, the surgeon did not know how close the rectum was despite visual and tactile cues. A more experienced surgeon would likely have sensed the approximate location and known that the rectum was near and that the tissue was too thick and pliable and would have stopped to reassess the situation before injury occurred.

ERRORS OF SITUATION AWARENESS
Surgical Video: Case 3

The video shows the surgeon excising endometriosis from the left pelvic sidewall, near the pelvic brim. The view seen is close and narrow. Laparoscopic scissors come into view and tip down, near a prominent ridge. The tips of the scissors close, and a surge of blood comes from the sidewall, darkening the lens and obscuring the view. The laparoscope is removed, cleaned, and placed back into the abdomen. A torrent of blood is seen coming from the left common iliac vein, and an immediate laparotomy is necessary.

In 2000, a Boeing 747 started its approach to takeoff during heavy rain caused by a typhoon. With poor visibility because of the rain, the flight crew did not see the parked construction equipment until the aircraft was too close, and the airplane broke up into pieces. The massive fire that resulted killed 79 passengers and 4 crew members.

The crew had attempted takeoff from a runway that had been closed for repairs. The accident investigation found that the flight crew had not reviewed the taxi route despite having all the relevant charts. The flight crew had also neglected to check 2 displays, which indicated that the aircraft was lined up on the wrong runway. Hurried by the imminent arrival of the typhoon and the poor weather conditions, the flight crew taxied toward disaster.

Situation awareness is defined as maintaining awareness of the operational environment and anticipating contingencies, or more simply "what's going on" and "what is likely to happen next."[11] Situation awareness involves vigilance, planning, time management, prioritizing tasks, and avoiding distractions. Although an integral part of a pilot's education, these principles are foreign to surgeons.

Visual, auditory, and touch perceptions are a necessary aspect of performing most tasks. Information from 2 or more senses (eg, during surgery, vision and touch) allows the brain to cross-validate perceptual information. Haptic perception, information from touch, is particularly useful during surgery. One disadvantage of laparoscopic surgery is the general loss of haptic perception, whereby the sense of the consistency and quality of tissue is diminished because of the interposition of rigid instruments between the tissue and hands, and therefore, the exquisite sensitivity of fingertip touch is lost entirely. In video 3, had the surgeon been able to feel for the pulsations of the common iliac artery, a sense of location would have been appreciated. Learning how to compensate for haptic deficits with visual information must occur with practice and over time.

Laparoscopic surgery eliminates binocular depth perception, making spatial orientation more difficult. In surgical case 3, had the surgeon pulled back the laparoscope to widen the angle of view, the general sense of where the major vessels were located would have been appreciated. Also, had the surgeon used the classically taught surgical technique, traction/countertraction to develop tissue planes, and used the scissors with tips up, injury to a major vessel might have been avoided.

ERRORS RELATED TO STRESS OR SLEEP DEPRIVATION
Surgical Video: Case 4

A 16-year-old girl with acute onset of pelvic pain is seen in the emergency room, and a sonogram finds a 2-cm simple cyst in the right ovary. The consulting gynecologist recommends laparoscopic evaluation because of the intensity of the pain. During a laparoscopic survey of the pelvis, the video shows normal ovaries and no pathologic conditions. The right ovary is braced against the right pelvic sidewall as a monopolar spatula is used to incise the ovary in an attempt to find the 2-cm cyst. Just then, the activated monopolar spatula slips to the pelvic sidewall, producing a steady stream of blood. The right common iliac vein has been lacerated.

The assistant instantly grasps the area in an attempt to stem the bleeding. However, the assistant's grasper has sharp teeth and a cutting edge, which tears a hole in the common iliac artery, and the pelvis is seen filling with blood. The surgeon spreads open the retroperitoneum, further tearing both the vein and the artery, and the stream of blood is now a flood. The surgeon attempts to control the bleeding with bipolar forceps, which at this point is futile. After many minutes that seem like hours, the video ends, and a laparotomy was performed. A vascular surgeon was called in to repair the damage. Because of the extensive damage, primary vessel repairs were not possible and grafting of both the right iliac artery and vein were necessary. However, the grafts subsequently fail. Reoperation and repeat grafting is performed, but these procedures also fail. The 16-year-old girl eventually requires below-the-knee amputation of her right leg.

In 1949, a raging forest fire threatened parts of central Montana, near a dry riverbank called Mann Gulch.[4] A crew of 15 smoke jumpers was flown ahead of the fire to put it out. High winds began fueling the fire, and, in an instant, the winds changed direction and started driving the fire toward the men. Fire now blocked the route of escape, and with the fire raging at their heels, the men panicked and started to run. The crew chief, Wag Dodge, realized that escape was hopeless and stopped running. He thought for a minute, took out a match, and set a fire directly in front of him. The small fire burned through the brush and quickly moved on, leaving a patch of scorched earth. He called to his men, telling them to do the same thing. However, 14 panicked men ran right past him and started up a nearby ridge. Wag stepped into the burnt area, lied down, and put a wet handkerchief over his face. The fire raged past him, but he was unhurt. He was the only survivor, and today, his method of escaping fire is taught to firefighters throughout the world.

Both surgical case 4 and the death of Mann Gulch firefighters illustrate reactions to stressful and frightening situations. The brain is hardwired to detect danger. Perceived patterns of danger are sent directly to the amygdala, the brain's early warning and emotional response center, where they are quickly processed unconsciously. A sense of danger triggers the "fight or flight" response, characterized by the activation of the sympathetic nervous system with the release of norepinephrine from nerve endings, which acts on the heart, blood vessels, respiratory centers, and other regions. Quickly, tachycardia and a state of arousal ensue. Attention is narrowed, a state likened to momentary autism.[6] Peripheral vision becomes restricted, and incoming information is selectively limited. All this happens unconsciously and quickly; see a snake, run, then feel fear. Running away, however, is not an option for the surgeon.

At some optimal level of stress or arousal, narrowing of attention enhances cognitive and physical performance. However, increasing levels of stress cause performance to decline quickly because other incoming information does not get processed, and errors may follow. This phenomenon is graphically illustrated by the Yerkes-Dodson law (**Fig. 4**).

In the Mann Gulch fire, had the firefighters stopped and followed Wag Dodge's lead, they all would have survived. Snap decisions made in the absence of expertise and experience (panic) can be devastatingly bad. Panic leads to a narrowing of thoughts; in this case, run for your life. Dodge was able to hold off these emotions, stop, and deliberately think about a novel solution to a dangerous threat. It saved his life. Surgical video 4 also clearly shows that the surgeon's and assistant's reactions were fueled by fear and panic. Even allowing for improper surgical technique, poor choice of instruments, improper use of the pelvic sidewall as a backstop, and the unfortunate injury to the iliac vein, a deliberate and thought-out response could have salvaged the situation. Pressure applied to the injured area with a 4 × 8 inches gauze (pushed down the umbilical cannula) would have limited blood loss. Performance of an immediate laparotomy through a midline incision while the nurses called for a vascular surgeon would have allowed full tamponade of the vessel until the surgeon arrived. This measured response would have resulted in no further injury, no need for vascular grafting, and no amputation of the girl's leg.

Perceptual learning is prevented by sleep deprivation because sleep is required for pattern consolidation in long-term memory. Fatigue and stress affect performance, even among highly skilled and experienced individuals. However, many surgeons are unwilling to recognize this fact. When presented with the statement "even when fatigued I perform effectively," 70% of the surgeons agreed with the statement compared with only 26% of pilots.[12] Chronically high concentrations of glucocorticoids associated with chronic stress can damage the memory (hippocampal) neurons and lead to memory disruption.

KNOWLEDGE-BASED ERRORS
Surgical Video: Case 5

A 25-year-old woman is admitted for laparoscopic surgery to determine the cause of chronic pelvic pain. The video shows the surgeon using an argon beam coagulator (ABC) to remove endometriosis on the peritoneum near the right pelvic sidewall. A venous plexus near the right uterosacral ligament begins to bleed briskly. Continued

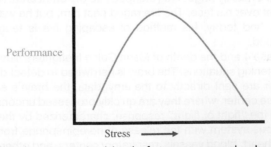

Fig. 4. Yerkes-Dodson law. An optimal level of stress or arousal enhances cognitive and physical performance. Increased levels of stress cause performance to decline quickly. *From* Parker WH, Johns A, Hellige J. Avoiding complications of laparoscopic surgery: lessons from cognitive science and crew resource management. J Minim Invasive Gynecol 2007;14(3):381; with permission.

use of the argon beam for several minutes has little effect on the bleeding. Suddenly, a surge of gas bubbles is seen coming from the right pelvic sidewall. At that moment, the woman dies on the operating table from an argon gas embolus to the heart.

Surgical Video: Case 6

A woman with chronic pelvic pain is admitted for a laparoscopic uterosacral nerve ablation. The video shows a bipolar Kleppinger forceps being used to grasp each uterosacral ligament. Current is applied, and diffuse blanching is seen surrounding the ligaments. The patient is discharged home the same day. After 2 days, the patient returns with an acute abdomen. At laparotomy, urine is found in the abdomen and both ureters are found to have been injured by thermal damage near the desiccated uterosacral ligaments. Reimplantation of both ureters into the bladder is necessary.

In 1997, John Denver, the singer and amateur pilot, was flying his newly built experimental airplane when it veered sharply to the right and plunged into Monterey Bay, killing him.[13] An investigation found that, before takeoff Denver had gotten falsely elevated fuel readings because of the tilt of the airplane on the ground. The airplane builder had also modified the original kit design and placed the fuel valve behind the pilot's left shoulder. So, to reach the fuel valve, Denver had to reach over his left shoulder with his right hand. This action caused Denver to brace himself with his right foot, causing him to step on the rudder pedal. The airplane veered to the right and spiraled into the ocean. Had Denver been familiar with the airplane and known how to properly gauge the fuel level, or had he been more accustomed to the awkward placement of the fuel valve, the crash could have been avoided.

Knowledge about the surgical instruments and energy sources that are used is imperative. The ABC forces argon gas through a nozzle tip at 6 to 8 L/min, carrying electric current to the tissue. Whereas carbon dioxide is highly soluble in blood (water) and relatively safe, argon is insoluble in blood and the gas bubbles remain in the circulation. With an open venous plexus, as the flow of argon gas increased the intra-abdominal pressure, argon was forced into the circulation. As gas collected in the heart, no blood could be effectively pumped back to the heart or brain, and death quickly ensued.

In addition, the ABC fulgurates just the surface of tissue and is not likely to be effective in controlling deep venous bleeding; it was a poor choice of instruments. Dissection of the ureters away from the vessels followed by application of clips, suture, or directed bipolar energy would have been more effective and would have had less risk.

In case 6, electrosurgery uses electric current to heat water molecules within the tissue. Rapidly increasing temperature, resulting from unmodulated or cutting current, causes water vapor to form within cells, causing subsequent explosion of the cells. Underlying cells are subject to less energy. Slower application of energy, as the result of modulated current, commonly called coagulation but properly called desiccation, causes denaturation of protein within cells. Because surface cells remain intact, they conduct heat to the underlying cells, which may also be injured. Adjacent thermal injury is usually not immediately apparent because it takes a few days for the cells to deteriorate and for the clinical signs and symptoms to become apparent.

Thermal injury to adjacent tissue may be reduced by using cutting current rather than coagulating current. Compression of the tissue with a grasping forceps before desiccation can reduce blood flow through the tissue and lessen the heat sink effect, whereby heat is removed from the treated area and carried to adjacent tissue. Pulsing of the energy on and off every few seconds allows the tissue to cool in the off cycle, reducing risk. Cool irrigation fluid used to bathe the adjacent tissue may also reduce inadvertent injury. Judicious dissection of structures and separation from adjacent tissue may also help to avoid inadvertent injury to nearby tissue during desiccation.

The deliberate study of energy sources and their proper use should be incorporated into every surgeon's education.

THE WRONG STUFF
Surgical Video: Case 7

A 36-year-old woman complains of pelvic pain, and a sonogram identifies small uterine myomas. The video of the laparoscopic surgery reveals no abnormalities of the pelvis. The surgeon, however, has invited a colleague to help him learn how to use the Nd:YAG laser. The surgeon focuses on a 1-cm nodule near the lower uterine segment, perhaps the fibroid that was seen during sonography. The nodule is grasped, and the laser is activated to remove the mass. The tissue appears tubular and easily stretches with traction. After a few minutes of stretching and cutting, the myoma starts to bleed profusely. A close view clearly shows this structure to be the ascending branch of the uterine artery. Apparently unable to stop the bleeding, laparotomy and hysterectomy are performed. Despite no clinically significant pathologic condition being seen, no one in the operating room questioned what the surgeons were doing.

In 1989, a commercial airliner was preparing for takeoff in a snowstorm but was delayed by an incoming plane. During the delay, the passengers noted accumulation of snow on the wings and reported this to the flight attendant. Without deicing the wings, the airplane tookoff and crashed just beyond the runway. Twenty-two of the 64 passengers and both pilots were killed in the crash. The flight attendant survived. When interviewed during an inquiry after the accident, she said that she had never been trained to question something that was the pilot's responsibility.[14]

Following a rash of airline crashes, the National Aeronautics and Space Administration organized an aviation conference in 1979. Investigation revealed that the causes of most airline accidents were not mechanical failure or lack of technical skill, but rather failures of interpersonal communication, decision making, and leadership.[15] After the conference, commercial airlines started intensive training programs (crew resource management) to change the behavior of cockpit crews. Authoritarian behavior by captains, termed the "Wrong Stuff," and lack of assertiveness by junior officers was no longer tolerated.[16] Role playing in emergency situations was instituted as part of mandatory training. Flight crews are now required to take periodic training in team building, decision-making strategies, situation awareness, and stress management. Mistakes are admitted, and critique is accepted objectively and nondefensively. Friendly, relaxed, and supportive crew interactions are encouraged. Conflicts of opinion are clearly stated and resolved using reasoned argument and appropriate evidence. Essential activities (flying the airplane) are maintained as information is collected and decisions are made. After a near miss, black box flight recorders are monitored to ensure that proper communication was maintained.

This transformation, along with important advances in computer systems, is responsible for a 99% reduction in the number of fatal crashes per 1 million departures, from 11.5 in 1970 to 0.2 in 2009.

Research shows that the best way to improve performance is to focus on mistakes. Dopamine neurons continually generate patterns based on experience. If a pattern is correct then the neurons produce a burst of dopamine, which is experienced as pleasure. If the neural patterns are incorrect then the neurons in the anterior cingulate cortex responsible for error detection generate a signal called the "oh, shit" circuit.[4] Mistakes cause the brain to revise its unconscious models. There are no shortcuts to this process, and successful training must accept, in a nonpunitive way, that errors will occur and emphasize the necessity of learning from one's mistakes.

After instituting a confidential, no-fault reporting system, the Federal Aviation Administration collected 6000 reports of errors and near-miss situations over 2 years. Although these practices will need to be modified for the operating room environment, consideration should be given to setting up similar required training courses, audio-tape reviews of operating room discussion, and no-fault reporting systems for surgeons, assistants, and staff.

Current technology exists to help prevent medical systems errors such as alerting physicians to abnormal test results, monitoring medication orders, and detecting drug incompatibilities or drug allergies. In the operating room, once surgery starts there are no automated safeguards. Recently, time-outs have been instituted at the beginning of the procedure so that the entire operating room team can verify the patient's name and go over the type of procedure, patient allergies, and any specific concerns such as the likelihood of significant blood loss. Some institutions have implemented checklists, which often include checking for the proper operative site, checking that the operating room team is aware of the patient's allergies, checking that antibiotics are given if indicated, and checking for significant medical conditions that may influence the surgical outcome.[17] In addition to avoiding obvious errors, these processes have been shown to build team communication. The fundamental premise is that a true team approach is safer and more efficient than the traditional pyramidal hierarchy in the operating room.

Again, the airline industry has shown us that this approach works. Most commercial airline pilots were trained in the military, where the culture of "captain of the ship" existed and was carried over to commercial airplanes. Crew resource management was used to break down these barriers and open communication so that other members of the crew could add expertise and knowledge. The surgeon, assistant, scrub nurse, circulating nurse, and anesthesiologist all view the same image on video monitors and can see the details of the ongoing procedure. Whereas the surgeon may be focused on one specific task at a time, others may be able to see potential problems and voice their concern. The paradigm of surgeon as the captain of the ship and sole source of knowledge needs to change, as it has among airline crews.

An example of the application of crew resource management to health care includes the following underlying principles: team responsibility for patients, belief in clinician fallibility, peer monitoring, and awareness of patient status. If, during monitoring of a situation, team members suspect an error in progress, they are instructed to ask a direct question or offer information. If a strong disagreement arises, third party involvement may be used to resolve the situation.[12] In surgical video of case 7, if someone had questioned what the surgeon was doing and why, the patient would not have been subjected to an unnecessary surgery that resulted in a laparotomy and hysterectomy and the surgeons would not have been subjected to a lawsuit.

ERRORS IN TRAINING

Both deliberate practice aimed at specific components of a task and actual experience are necessary to achieve high levels of performance. For chess masters, professional musicians, and professional athletes it takes about 5000 hours of deliberate learning and practice to become an expert. A minimum of 10 years of intense involvement, accumulating the necessary knowledge and experience in the instinctive portion of the brain, is crucial to reach a high level of performance in all these fields.[18] The same is likely true for expert surgeons.

Assume that a challenging laparoscopic procedure takes about 2 hours. In a busy gynecologic practice, 2 challenging laparoscopic procedures a week might be performed. At that rate, the surgeon would accumulate 200 hours of experience a year and become an expert after 25 years. Even with 5 challenging cases per week, it would take 10 years to achieve this level of experience. Approximately 630,000 hysterectomies are performed annually by 32,000 practicing gynecologists in the United States.[19] On average then, most gynecologists will perform less than 2 procedures per month. Approximately 59,000 of these hysterectomies are performed laparoscopically, so experience with laparoscopic hysterectomy is significantly less.

Again, the airline industry has something to teach us. To get an entry-level job as a first officer for a commercial airline, about 1000 hours of flying experience is necessary. The first officers are required to complete 40 hours of training in the appropriate aircraft simulator before they can fly. When a first officer upgrades to captain, 3500 hours of flying experience plus another 25 hours in the simulator are required. Furthermore, every 6 months the pilots must go through simulator flying to demonstrate competence. Critically important is that pilots are put into simulated emergency situations (loss of an engine), in which danger is imminent, stress is created, and the pilots need to navigate their way out. Performance is judged, and errors are reviewed, so the pilots can learn from this experience. When a problem that has never been experienced before is encountered, the dopamine neurons have no idea what to do. Here it is essential to tune out feelings; deliberate calm requires conscious effort. These situations also present an overload of information. The pilot must minimize distractions, think about what to think about, and prioritize tasks. Practicing all this allows pilots to better control the stress response during a real emergency. People who are more rational in emergency situations do not perceive emotion less; they just regulate it better.[4]

However, simulation for laparoscopic surgery is far behind flight simulation. Most surgical simulators are limited to normal anatomy and simple skill sets and cannot simulate abnormal anatomy, emergencies, or complications.[20,21] We want surgeons to make mistakes. We know that is how we learn best. We just do not want patients to be subject to these mistakes. Realistic simulators are the proven way to properly train surgeons.[22] Computer power and technology exist, but major funding will be needed to develop simulators and teaching modules for surgical training programs.

Distributed practice is usually better than massed practice; it is more productive to practice 2 hours a day for 50 days than to practice 10 hours a day for 5 days. In addition, it is usually better to learn in the same context or environment in which performance will take place. Challenges that lie just beyond the level of competence are most effective for continuing to build expertise.

SUMMARY

Deliberate accumulation of knowledge and experience must be acquired during residency training and for many years afterward. Many hours of practice in simulated situations and actual surgery are necessary to acquire the instinctual pattern recognition in long-term memory. Over time, this knowledge becomes instinctive and effortless, and skill level increases. Surgeons should understand that deliberate thinking is predominantly important until enough experience accrues for educated, instinctive thinking to be helpful. Specific attention should be directed toward learning pelvic anatomy, proper surgical techniques, proper function, and use of surgical instruments and energy sources. Managing surgical emergencies and complications can be taught by simulation, and efforts should be made to develop this area to enhance surgical training. We cannot escape the fact that we are humans, with all the inherent strengths and frailties of our species. Further understanding of cognitive issues as they relate to the performance of surgery may help improve quality of care and patient safety.

REFERENCES

1. Way LW, Stewart L, Gantert W, et al. Causes and prevention of laparoscopic bile duct injuries: analysis of 252 cases from a human factors and cognitive psychology perspective. Ann Surg 2003;237:460–9.
2. Parker W, Johns A, Helige J. Avoiding complications of laparoscopic surgery: lessons from cognitive science and crew resource management. J Minim Invasive Gynecol 2007;14:379–88.
3. Norretranders T. The user illusion: cutting consciousness down to size. New York: Viking; 1998.
4. Leher J. How we decide. New York: Mariner Books; 2010.
5. Margolis H. Patterns, thinking and cognition: a theory of judgment. Chicago: University of Chicago Press; 1990.
6. Gladwell M. Blink: the power of thinking without thinking. New York: Little Brown; 2005.
7. Croskerry P, Sinclair D. Emergency medicine: a practice prone to error? CJEM 2001;3:271–6.
8. Pascual-Leone A, Torres F. Plasticity of the sensorimotor cortex representation of the reading finger in Braille readers. Brain 1993;116:39–52.
9. Kellman P. Learning, motivation, and emotion. In: Gallistel R, editor. Stevens' handbook of experimental psychology. Hoboken (NJ): John Wiley and Sons; 2002. p. 267.
10. Norman D. Things that make us smart. Reading (MA): Perseus Books; 1993.
11. Singh H, Petersen LA, Thomas EJ. Understanding diagnostic errors in medicine: a lesson from aviation. Qual Saf Health Care 2006;15:159–64.
12. Pizzi L, Goldfarb N, Nash D. Crew resource management and its applicability in medicine. In: Markowitz A, editor. AHRQ evidence report/technology assessment. Rockville (MD): Agency for Healthcare Research and Quality. Number 43 (AHRQ Publication 01-E058); 2001. p. 505–13.
13. Tognazzini B. When interfaces kill: what really happened to John Denver. Available at: http://www.asktog.com/columns/027InterfacesThatKill.html. 1999. Accessed July 7, 2010.
14. Hamman WR. The complexity of team training: what we have learned from aviation and its applications to medicine. Qual Saf Health Care 2004;13(S1):i72–9.
15. Cooper G, White M, Lauber J, editors. Resource management on the flightdeck: proceedings of a NASA/industry workshop (NASA CP-2120). Moffett Field (CA): NASA-Ames Research Center; 1980.
16. Helmreich RL, Merritt AC, Wilhelm JA. The evolution of Crew Resource Management training in commercial aviation. Int J Aviat Psychol 1999;9:19–32.
17. Gwande A. The checklist manifesto. New York: Metropolitan Book; 2010.
18. Ericsson KA. Deliberate practice and the acquisition and maintenance of expert performance in medicine and related domains. Acad Med 2004;79:S70–81.
19. Farquhar C, Steiner C. Hysterectomy rates in the United States 1990–1997. Obstet Gynecol 2002;99:229–34.
20. Hasson HM. Core competency in laparoendoscopic surgery. JSLS 2006;10:16–20.
21. Hart R, Doherty DA, Karthigasu K, et al. The value of virtual reality-simulator training in the development of laparoscopic surgical skills. J Minim Invasive Gynecol 2006;13:126–33.
22. Guerlain S, Green K, LaFollette M, et al. Improving surgical pattern recognition through repetitive viewing of video clips. IEEE Trans Syst Man Cybern A Syst Hum 2004;34(no. 6):705.

Postoperative Neuropathy in Gynecologic Surgery

Amber D. Bradshaw, MD, Arnold P. Advincula, MD*

KEYWORDS

• Postoperative neuropathy • Nerve injury
• Postoperative complications

The development of a postoperative neuropathy is a rare complication that can be devastating to the patient. In a study of 1210 patients who underwent major pelvic surgery, the rate of postoperative neuropathy was found to be 1.9%.[1] Most cases of postoperative neuropathy are caused by improper patient positioning and the incorrect placement of surgical retractors. To fully understand the pathophysiology of postoperative neuropathy, the nerves that are at greatest risk of injury during gynecologic surgery will be presented through a series of vignettes. Suggestions for protection of each nerve will be provided.

Before embarking on a discussion of postoperative neuropathy, it is important to review a practical working classification of nerve injuries. In Seddon's classification system, there are three types of injury: neurapraxia, axonotmesis, and neurotmesis.[2] Knowing the classification system can aid in counseling patients regarding their prognosis and treatment options.

A mild injury to a nerve may cause a conduction block across a small portion of the affected nerve. This type of injury is called neurapraxia and is caused by external compression to the nerve.[3] This creates a disruption of the blood supply, which damages the nerve. This type of injury affects motor fibers more than sensory fibers. Recovery can take weeks or months and depends on how quickly the nerve fibers can remyelinate the segment that has been damaged.

A more severe injury to the nerve results in damage to the axon of the nerve, while maintaining preservation of the supporting Schwann cells. This type of injury is called axonotmesis and is caused by profound compression or traction on the nerve.[2] Both motor and sensory fibers can be affected as well as autonomic function. Even though the axon of the nerve is disrupted, regeneration is usually complete, because the supporting Schwann cells remain intact. The recovery time for axonotmesis is much longer than neurapraxia.

University of Central Florida College of Medicine, Center for Specialized Gynecology, Florida Hospital, Celebration Health, 410 Celebration Place, Suite 302, Celebration, FL 34747, USA
* Corresponding author.
E-mail address: arnold.advincula.md@flhosp.org

Obstet Gynecol Clin N Am 37 (2010) 451–459
doi:10.1016/j.ogc.2010.05.008
0889-8545/10/$ – see front matter © 2010 Elsevier Inc. All rights reserved.

obgyn.theclinics.com

The most severe injury is a complete interruption of the nerve and supporting structures. This nerve injury is called neurotmesis and is caused by transection or ligation of the nerve. Because both the nerve and supporting structures have been affected, neurotmesis has a poor prognosis for complete recovery. The necessary treatment is usually surgery to reconnect the two nerve ends.[2]

CASE 1

A 45-year-old Gravida (G) 5 Para (P) 5 (G5P5) presented with stage 3 pelvic organ prolapse. She was scheduled for a robot-assisted laparoscopic sacrocolpopexy. She was placed in dorsal lithotomy position, and shoulder braces were used to keep her from sliding on the table during steep Trendelenburg. As soon as the patient recovered from anesthesia, she complained of right hand numbness. On postoperative day number 1, a wrist drop was noted.

CASE 2

A 24-year-old G1 presented to the emergency room with abdominal pain and was found to be in hypovolemic shock. It was determined that the patient had a ruptured ectopic pregnancy, and she was taken immediately to the operating room. She underwents a laparotomy and left salpingectomy. During surgery, she was in supine position with her arms placed on arm boards. After 5 U of blood, she was stable and taken to the floor for recovery. On postoperative day number 1, she complained of pain and numbness to her left hand. On examination, there was significant weakness to the left lower arm and hand.

BRACHIAL PLEXUS INJURY

Case 1 and 2 represent two different mechanisms for developing a brachial plexus injury. The brachial plexus is made up of nerves from C5 to T1. These nerves course beneath the clavicle after branching out from the spinal cord. They then enter the arm medial to the humeral head. Usually the nerve plexus is protected by these bones. However, the structural relationship between the two can make the nerves more susceptible to stretch or compression injuries against the hard surface of the bone.

In the operating room, brachial plexus injuries can occur from several etiologies. The first is from the use of shoulder braces as seen in case 1. Often shoulder braces are used during laparoscopic surgery to prevent the patient from sliding on the operating room table (**Fig. 1**). This is a common issue when the patient is placed in steep Trendelenburg position. When shoulder braces are used, correct placement is important to prevent injury. If the shoulder brace is placed too lateral while the patient is in Trendelenburg position, a stretch injury can occur. Upward force on the shoulder by the brace is opposed by a downward gravitational force on the patient. These two opposing forces cause the brachial plexus to be stretched. General anesthesia tends to enhance this injury by creating increased joint mobility, especially when muscle relaxants are used. The shoulder brace also can cause an injury when placed too proximal to the neck. This causes a compression injury, because the brace presses the brachial plexus against the first rib.[4]

Correct placement of shoulder braces can help decrease the risk of a postoperative brachial plexus injury. The brace should be placed over the acromioclavicular joint, thereby avoiding a location that is too medial or lateral on the shoulder. Even with perfect positioning, however, a nerve injury can still occur. Finding an alternative to using the shoulder brace is a better option in reducing the risk of brachial plexus injury.

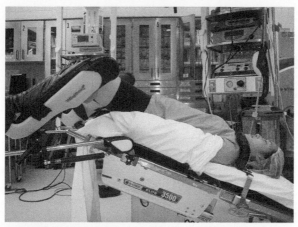

Fig. 1. Incorporation of shoulder braces during steep Trendelenburg. (*Courtesy of* Amber D. Bradshaw and Arnold P. Advinculala; with permission.)

Some physicians use bean bags or gel pads. Another alternative is using an egg crate foam mattress pad on top of the operating room draw sheets (**Fig. 2**). When placed against the patient's bare back, the drag coefficient, created by the weight of the patient and the pad, prevents the patient from slipping on the table during steep Trendelenburg.

Another situation where a brachial plexus injury can occur is demonstrated in case 2. Improper positioning of the upper extremities on arm boards places the patient at increased risk for a brachial plexus injury during surgery. The brachial plexus is at risk for a stretch or compression injury, as it runs caudal to the humeral head.[5] This can occur if for an extended period of time the arm is abducted greater than 90° from the body (**Fig. 3**). Inspecting the position of the arms on the arm boards before each surgery can reduce the risk of a brachial plexus injury. The arm boards may have been placed by the anesthesiologist or operating room staff and could be overlooked by a busy surgeon. An alternative to arm boards would be to tuck the arms at

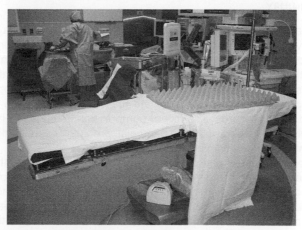

Fig. 2. Operating room set up with egg crate foam mattress padding on top of draw sheet. (*Courtesy of* Amber D. Bradshaw and Arnold P. Advincula; with permission.)

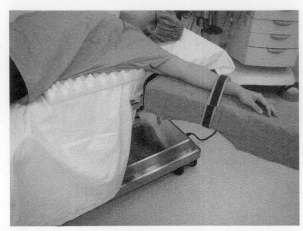

Fig. 3. Upper extremity abducted greater than 90° on arm board. (*Courtesy of* Amber D. Bradshaw and Arnold P. Advincula; with permission.)

the patient's side. Optimal positioning for tucking the arms will be addressed later. The symptoms of brachial plexus injury are variable. They range from slight numbness and tingling in the arm to the inability to move the arm. A characteristic wrist drop also may be observed.

CASE 3

A 46-year-old G1P1 presented with menorrhagia and a large fibroid uterus. She underwent a robot-assisted total laparoscopic hysterectomy and was placed in dorsal lithotomy position with her arms tucked at her sides. The surgery was prolonged due to the size and number of uterine fibroids. As the surgical drapes were removed, it was noted that the patient's left arm had slipped out of the tucked position and was resting on the metal rail of the operating room table. As the anesthesia wore off, she complained of numbness and weakness of the fourth and fifth fingers of her right hand.

ULNAR NERVE INJURY

The patient in case 3 represents an ulnar nerve injury. The ulnar nerve is located in the olecranon groove as it crosses the elbow. This groove is located posteriorly between the medial condyle of the humerus and the olecranon process of the ulna. In the olecranon groove, the ulnar nerve can be susceptible to injury, as it is only covered by minimal soft tissue. Compression of the ulnar nerve can occur in the operating room from incorrect positioning when the arms are tucked at the patient's side or when they are placed on arm boards. The risk of compression is related to how the lower arm is placed when in these positions. In particular, pronation or supination of the forearm is important depending on which position is used.

During laparoscopic surgery, a patient's arms often are tucked at the sides. This allows the surgeon to stand further up the table. Incorrect positioning of the forearm, when the arms are tucked, can lead to a compression injury of the ulnar nerve. When the forearm is supinated, the olecranon process is located posteromedially. This supinated position places the ulnar nerve at the greatest risk of injury. If the drawsheet loosens and the arm migrates down against the edge of the operating room table, the ulnar nerve can be compressed. For this reason, it is important for the surgeon to make sure that the forearm is in the pronated position before the arm is tucked at the patient's side (**Fig. 4**). This position will rotate the olecranon groove both outward and lateral, protecting the ulnar nerve from compression against the operating room table. Foam padding also can be placed at the elbow before the arms are tucked to add extra protection to the ulnar nerve.

Another situation where the ulnar nerve is at risk is during laparotomy. For an abdominal procedure, the patient's arms are usually placed on arm boards. Below the elbow, the ulnar nerve is unprotected and at risk for injury by incorrect positioning of the forearm on an arm board. If the forearm is pronated on the arm board, the ulnar nerve can be compressed between the arm board and the boney floor of the cubital tunnel. To decrease the risk of nerve injury, the surgeon should ensure the forearm is supinated before being placed on the arm board. Again, padding around the elbow can be used to protect the ulnar nerve from compression.

An ulnar nerve neuropathy presents with paresthesia of the fourth and fifth digit and the ulnar third of the hand. If the motor component of the nerve is affected, a claw hand may develop. This is caused by the fourth and fifth digits being hyperextended by the unopposed long extensors and the second and third digit being hyperflexed by the unopposed long flexors. Atrophy of the interosseous muscles also can occur.[5]

CASE 4

A 65-year-old G5P5 presented with stage 3 pelvic organ prolapse. She underwent a total vaginal hysterectomy, uterosacral ligament suspension, and anterior and posterior colporrhaphy. During the surgery, she was placed in the dorsal lithotomy position in candy cane stirrups. On postoperative day number 1, she complained of weakness in her lower extremities and had difficulty getting out of bed or climbing stairs.

CASE 5

A 45-year-old G2P2 presented with a history of stage 4 endometriosis and pelvic pain. She underwent a total abdominal hysterectomy, bilateral salpingo-oophorectomy, and lysis of adhesions through a Pfannenstiel skin incision. A self-retaining retractor was used for exposure. On postoperative day number 1, the patient complained of paresthesia over the medial aspect of the right thigh and knee. She also exhibited a weakness in her right leg.

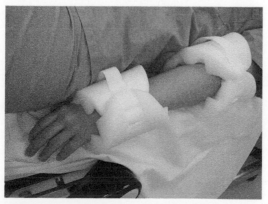

Fig. 4. Proper placement of the tucked upper extremity in pronated position at the patient's side. (*Courtesy of* Amber D. Bradshaw and Arnold P. Advincula; with permission.)

FEMORAL NERVE INJURY

Case 4 and 5 represent two mechanisms for sustaining an injury to the femoral nerve. The largest branch of the lumbar plexus is the femoral nerve. It courses between the psoas and iliacus muscles in the abdomen. After coursing underneath the inguinal ligament, it then enters the thigh. This anatomy makes the femoral nerve susceptible to injury at several points along its course.

During a laparotomy, self-retaining retractors often are used for exposure. The incidence of femoral nerve injury with self-retaining retractors has been reported to be 7% to 12%.[6] The femoral nerve is at risk for compression from the retractor blades in two ways. The first is from the retractor blades resting directly on the psoas muscle. This compresses the femoral nerve as it passes underneath the psoas. The risk of compression increases when excessively long retractor blades are used. Thin patients are at a greater risk because of a shorter distance between the anterior abdominal wall and the psoas muscle. A second way self-retaining retractor blades can cause compression of the femoral nerve is from directly retracting the psoas muscle laterally. If this occurs, the femoral nerve is compressed between the retractor blade and the boney pelvic sidewall. This type of injury is more likely with a large Pfannenstiel skin incision, because it allows more lateral placement of the retractor blades.[6] It is important for the surgeon to carefully consider the retractor he or she uses during abdominal surgery. If a self-retaining retractor is used in a thin patient, the shortest blades that accommodate the patient's anterior abdominal wall should be employed. Also, rolled laparotomy sponges should be placed between the retractor and the abdominal wall. This creates more space between the retractor blade and the psoas muscle. If the surgery becomes lengthy, releasing the retractors intermittently can reduce the risk of compression to the femoral nerve. An alternative to traditional self-retaining retractors are disposable self-retaining retractors. These retractors provide uniform exposure without the use of blades. Thus there is no risk of compression to the femoral nerve.[7]

The femoral nerve also can be injured during lithotomy position in candy cane stirrups as in case 4. This is caused by excessive hip flexion or extreme abduction and external rotation of the thigh (**Fig. 5**). These positions cause the femoral nerve to be angulated and compressed against the inguinal ligament. The longer the patient is in these extreme positions, the more likely an injury is to occur. Compression of the

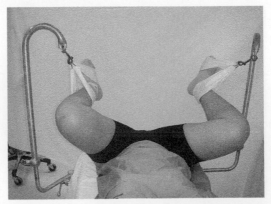

Fig. 5. Hyperflexion of hips while in candy cane stirrups. (*Courtesy of* Amber D. Bradshaw and Arnold P. Advincula; with permission.)

femoral nerve also can be caused by surgical assistants leaning against the patient's inner thigh during surgery.[4] To reduce the risk of femoral neuropathy, it is important for the surgeon to check the patient's lower extremity positioning when placing a patient in candy cane stirrups. The surgeon should make sure the thigh is not overly abducted or rotated and that the hip is not hyperflexed beyond 80° or 90°. It is also important to educate surgical assistants about the danger of leaning on the patient's lower extremity during retraction.

A femoral neuropathy can cause paresthesias of the thigh and leg and an inability to flex at the hip or to extend at the knee. It also can cause a decreased or absent patellar reflex. Postoperative classic symptoms are falling when trying to get out of bed and the inability to climb stairs.

CASE 6

A 42-year-old G4P4 presented with menorrhagia refractory to medical management. She underwent a total vaginal hysterectomy and was placed in dorsal lithotomy position in candy cane stirrups. After the procedure, she was noted to have a foot drop and paresthesia of the lateral lower leg and dorsum of the foot.

COMMON PERONEAL NERVE INJURY

The patient in case 6 represents a common peroneal injury. The common peroneal nerve courses laterally across the knee joint before it wraps around the fibular head to enter the lower leg. With its close proximity to the bone and little superficial protection, the common peroneal nerve is vulnerable to injury. Compression of the common peroneal nerve can occur in the operating room from incorrect positioning when candy cane stirrups are used. If the patient's knee and lower leg are allowed to press against the hard surface of the candy cane stirrups, the common peroneal nerve can be pressed against the fibular head. It is important to inspect the lower leg when the patient is placed in candy cane stirrups. The knee or lower leg should not be in contact with the stirrup. Padding of the knee also can be used for extra protection against injury.

An injury to the common peroneal nerve can cause a paresthesia of the lateral lower leg and dorsum of the foot. If the motor fibers are affected, weakness of the ankle extensors and foot dorsiflexors can occur. This may cause a characteristic foot drop.

CASE 7

A 34-year-old G3P3 presented with dysmenorrhea and was found to have adenomyosis on magnetic resonance imaging (MRI). She underwent a total abdominal hysterectomy through a Pfannenstiel skin incision. At the time the fascia was closed, it was noted that the incision extended laterally beyond the rectus muscles. On postoperative day number 1, the patient noted a sharp pain at her incision that radiated to the pubic bone. She also noted a numbness of her mons pubis and labia majora.

ILIOHYPOGASTRIC AND ILIOINGUINAL NERVE INJURY

Case 7 illustrates an injury to nerves within the abdominal wall. The iliohypogastric and ilioinguinal nerves arise from T12-L1 and are at risk for injury during abdominal surgery. These nerves run laterally through the head of the psoas muscle and penetrate the transversus abdominis muscle before entering the anterior abdominal wall.[6] These nerves are usually not injured during gynecologic surgery unless a Pfannenstiel skin incision is brought laterally beyond the edge of the rectus abdominis muscles. This wide incision puts the edge of the fascia in close proximity to these nerve branches. Damage to the nerve can occur from direct injury, incorporation during the fascial closure, or scar tissue formation after surgery. To decrease the risk of injury to the iliohypogastric and ilioinguinal nerves, the width of the Pfannenstiel incision should be kept within the rectus abdominis muscles. If the surgeon finds more exposure into the abdomen is needed, a Cherney or Maylard incision can be used. Performing these procedures laparoscopically also will decrease the risk of this nerve injury. During laparoscopic surgery, trocar sites are typically placed away from these nerve branches. Symptoms of an iliohypogastric or ilioinguinal nerve injury are a sharp pain and a burning sensation at the incision. There also can be a paresthesia over the mons pubis, labia, or inner thigh.

CASE 8

A 40-year-old woman presented with pelvic pain and a history of stage 4 endometriosis. She had failed multiple medical therapies and underwent an abdominal hysterectomy with resection of endometriosis, enterolysis, and ureterolysis. On postoperative day number 1, the patient complained of groin pain and numbness over her anterior thigh.

GENITOFEMORAL NERVE INJURY

The genitofemoral nerve arises from L1-2. It runs on top of the psoas muscle before splitting near the inguinal ligament. Because of the location of the genitofemoral nerve relative to the psoas muscle, it is also at risk for a compression injury during laparotomy. Compression of the genitofemoral nerve can occur when using self-retaining retractors. To reduce the risk of this nerve injury, the same precautions can be taken that were noted earlier when the femoral nerve was discussed. Another cause of injury to the genitofemoral nerve is inadvertent transection during a retroperitoneal dissection. A genitofemoral nerve injury can result in a paresthesia over the anterior thigh below the inguinal ligament. Groin pain also can occur.

CASE 9

Six years after a total vaginal hysterectomy, a 46-year-old G6P6 presented with symptomatic pelvic organ prolapse and stress urinary incontinence. She underwent a sacrospinous ligament suspension, anterior and posterior colporrhaphy, and transvaginal tape procedure. The patient was placed in dorsal lithotomy position in candy cane stirrups. After the procedure, she complained of paresthesias of the anterolateral thigh.

LATERAL FEMORAL CUTANEOUS NERVE INJURY

The lateral femoral cutaneous nerve arises from L2-4 and courses over the iliacus. It then runs underneath the inguinal ligament near the anterior superior iliac spine. This nerve can be injured in the operating room during lithotomy position. A compression injury can occur from excessive flexion of the hip. Checking the lower extremity position before surgery will help resolve any excessive flexion of the hip. An injury to the lateral femoral cutaneous nerve causes a sensory loss over the anterolateral thigh from the inguinal ligament to the knee.

SUMMARY

Postoperative neuropathies are rare but serious complications of surgery. Most nerve injuries occur from incorrect patient positioning or placement of self-retaining retractors used in the operating room. Understanding the anatomy of the nerves and how this neuroanatomical relationship can contribute to a compression or stretch injury is important to prevent this complication. Before each surgery, the surgeon should always check the position of every patient's upper and lower extremities. It is also important for the surgeon to choose the right retractor for the patient's anatomy. When these steps are followed, the risk of postoperative neuropathy will be decreased, and patient safety will be significantly improved.

REFERENCES

1. Cardosi RJ, Cox CS, Hoffman MS. Postoperative neuropathies after major pelvic surgery. Obstet Gynecol 2002;100(2):240–4.
2. Dumitru D. Electrodiagnostic medicine. Philadelphia: Hanley & Belfus; 1995. p. 350–2.
3. Campbell WW. Diagnosis and management of common compression and entrapment neuropathies. Neurol Clin 1997;15(3):549–67.
4. Winfree CJ, Kline DJ. Intraoperative positioning nerve injuries. Surg Neurol 2005; 63:5–18.
5. Dornette WHL. Identifying, moving, and positioning the patient. In: Dornette WHL, editor. Legal issues in anesthesia practice. Philadelphia: FA Davis; 1991. p. 113–24.
6. Irvin W, Andersen W, Taylor P, et al. Minimizing the risk of neurologic injury in gynecologic surgery. Obstet Gynecol 2004;103(2):374–82.
7. Pelosi MA II, Pelosi MA III. Self-retaining abdominal retractor for minilaparotomy. Obstet Gynecol 2000;96:775–8.

Hollow Viscus Injury During Surgery

Howard T. Sharp, MD*, Carolyn Swenson, MD

KEYWORDS

- Bladder injury • Ureter injury • Gastrointestinal injury
- Complications • Gynecologic surgery • Laparoscopy
- Cystoscopy

Reproductive tract surgery carries a risk of injury to the bladder, ureter, and gastrointestinal (GI) tract. This is due to several factors including close surgical proximity of these organs, disease processes that can distort anatomy, delayed mechanical and energy effects, and the inability to directly visualize organ surfaces. The informed consent process involves discussing potential damage to these structures. Ideally, injury to these organs is recognized and repaired intraoperatively. Unfortunately, these injuries are often the not immediately recognized due to the previously mentioned challenges. The purpose of this article is to review strategies to prevent, recognize, and repair injury to the GI and urinary tract during gynecologic surgery.

URINARY TRACT INJURY

The incidence of ureter and bladder injury during major gynecologic surgery is estimated to be 2 to 6 per 1000 cases and 3 to 12 per 1000 cases respectively.[1,2] A recent prospective study of 839 hysterectomies, however, demonstrated a much higher injury rate of 1.8% (N = 15) for ureter injury, and 2.9% (N = 24) for bladder injury.[3] Of urinary tract injuries, bladder injuries are up to 15 times more likely to be recognized intraoperatively compared with ureter injuries.[4] This is likely because of the ability to visualize the exposed Foley catheter in bladder injury cases.

BLADDER INJURY
Prevention and Detection of Bladder Injury

Laparoscopically assisted vaginal hysterectomy and bladder neck suspension surgery have the highest incidence of bladder injury, with rates of 2.8% and 1.9% respectively.[5,6] In a review of over 1300 articles citing complication during laparoscopy, electrosurgical dissection was the leading cause of bladder injury.[7] Intraoperative recognition of bladder injury occurred in a minority of cases.

Department of Obstetrics and Gynecology, University of Utah Health Sciences Center, Room 2B-200, 1900 East, 30 North, Salt Lake City, UT 84132, USA
* Corresponding author.
E-mail address: howard.sharp@hsc.utah.edu

Obstet Gynecol Clin N Am 37 (2010) 461–467
doi:10.1016/j.ogc.2010.05.004
0889-8545/10/$ – see front matter © 2010 Elsevier Inc. All rights reserved.

Injury prevention starts with understanding risk factors. Risk factors for bladder injury include: endometriosis, infection, bladder overdistention, and adhesions from previous surgery, which may pull the bladder to a more superior location than anticipated. Endometriosis and adhesions both alter tissue planes. For example, during hysterectomy with altered tissue planes, it is important to use sharp dissection while dissecting the bladder away from the lower uterine segment. The use of a blunt object such as a sponge stick with pressure will result in tearing at the site of least resistance, which may be the bladder rather than the fascial tissue plane. It is also important to recognize anatomy properly. If scarring has distorted the bladder anatomy significantly, the bladder can be filled with saline or water, in a retrograde fashion through a Foley catheter to better decipher its boundaries. During laparoscopic surgery, bladder overdistention can be avoided with the use of a Foley catheter. Lateral trocar placement rather than suprapubic placement will further lessen the risk of bladder injury.

Bladder injury is sometimes obvious, such as when the Foley catheter is seen or felt, when there is gas in the Foley catheter collection bag, or when a gush of urine is seen in the operative field. Continuing hematuria is also suggestive but not diagnostic of urinary tract injury, as transient hematuria is common as a result of urinary tract manipulation during surgery. Signs and symptoms of bladder injury may often be subtle, especially in the case of thermal injury, which usually does not manifest fully until several days later. When such risk factors are present, careful inspection of the bladder is recommended.

Management of Bladder Injury

There are two key concepts to consider when a bladder injury is discovered. One is to close the entirety of the defect. The other is to assess whether there is ureter involvement. To close the defect, the mucosa and muscularis are closed using a delayed absorbable suture in a running fashion. Most surgeons choose to close the bladder in two layers, placing a reinforcing layer through the serosa. The suture line can be assessed for leaking by placing 300 mL of dilute indigo or methylene blue dye in normal saline or water, retrograde into the bladder through a Foley catheter. The ureters should be assessed for patency. This can be done by feeding a ureteral catheter into both ureters through the defect (before it is closed), or cytoscopically after the defect is closed. Alternatively, indigo carmine (20 mg) may be given intravenously to ensure dye is observed to efflux from both ureters. Methylene blue should not be given intravenously because of the risk of methylhemoglobinemia.

There are differing opinions as to how long a Foley catheter should remain in place after bladder injury. If the injury occurred in the non-]dependent portion of the bladder (bladder dome), bladder drainage for 4 to 7 days is adequate. If the injury is located in the dependant portion of the bladder, such as the trigone, a catheter should remain for 7 to 14 days. Small defects less than 1 cm that were not the result of electrosurgical trauma may not need to be repaired, as spontaneous healing usually occurs. Laparoscopic repair may be performed in the case of smaller injury with adequate surgical expertise and adequate exposure, as long as the ureters and bladder neck are not compromised.[8]

URETER INJURY
Prevention and Detection of Ureter Injury

There are two common locations for ureteral injury. The most common site of injury is at the level of the uterine artery, which may be located within 1 cm of the ureter. The second most common site for ureteral injury is at the pelvic brim, where the ureter crosses the iliac vessels before it descends into the pelvis along the medial leaf of the broad ligament. The pelvic brim location is particularly vulnerable when performing oophorectomy while clamping across the infundibular ligament.

The mechanism of ureteral injury may be transection, crush injury, devascularization during tissue dissection, or damage with adjacent thermal energy while gaining hemostasis. Unfortunately, ureter injuries usually are not diagnosed intraoperatively.[7] The usual time to diagnosis of the postoperative patient with ureter injury is between postoperative days 2 and 7, but ureter injury has been diagnosed and reported as late as 33 days after surgery.[9] Patients often present with symptoms of abdominal pain, fever, hematuria, flank pain, and peritonitis. Leukocytosis is common.

One method to avoid injuring the ureter is to perform a retroperitoneal dissection of the ureter before clamping tissue pedicles. This is especially helpful in cases of significant endometriosis, adnexal masses, and fibroids that push into the pelvic sidewall. To perform this, the round ligament should be ligated as laterally as possible. The avascular perirectal and perivessicle spaces may be developed. The ureter is found along the medial aspect of the broad ligament. In cases where it is difficult to see the ureter, it usually can be palpated easily between the thumb and middle finger, as a nonpulsatile, rubbery organ. As the ureter descends from the pelvic brim toward the bladder, it becomes more difficult to follow, particularly as it disappears into the web of fascia near the bladder. Complete ureterolysis, which is usually not necessary except for cases of significant anatomic distortion, should be performed by a surgeon well trained in this procedure.

Management of Ureter Injury

If ureter injury is suspected, patency can be evaluated by performing a cystotomy or by cystoscopy. If cystotomy is used, it should be made at the bladder dome. The ureters then are identified, and a ureteral stent is fed through both ureteral orifices to evaluate for obstruction. If cystoscopy is performed, visualizing dye efflux or stent placement may be performed. A surgeon who is familiar with these techniques should perform these assessments. Although many gynecologists are credentialed and experienced in these procedures, if there is doubt about the presence of an injury after initial evaluation, a urologist should be consulted intraoperatively or as soon as diagnosed. In most cases, percutaneous or cystoscopic stenting techniques can be used.[10] Laparotomy usually is performed to repair by end-to-end anastomosis or reimplantation into the bladder, although in experienced hands, repair may be performed laparoscopically.[11]

Routine Cystoscopy

The use of routine cystoscopy after major gynecologic surgery has been embraced by some surgeons, yet it remains controversial because of the lack of high-quality studies to demonstrate clear cost benefits and diagnostic accuracy. In a systematic review of 47 larger published series (more than 500 cases per study), the use of routine cystoscopy resulted in an intraoperative diagnosis of ureteric injury in 89% (47 of 53) of cases, and bladder injury in 95% (59 of 62) of cases.[12] Comparatively, without cystoscopy, 7% (21 of 305) and 43% (105 of 450) of ureter and bladder injuries, respectively, were diagnosed intraoperatively. In a prospective study of 839 patients undergoing hysterectomy, 39 (4.3%) patients sustained a urinary tract injury, 97.4% of whom were diagnosed intraoperatively with the use of routine cystoscopy.[3]

The American College of Obstetricians and Gynecologists has recommended that cystoscopy be performed intraoperatively after all prolapse or incontinence surgery during which the bladder or ureters may be at risk of injury (level C recommendation, US Preventative Task Force).[13]

GI INJURY

Combined data show GI injury during gynecologic surgery occurs in between 0.05% and 0.33% of cases.[14] Intraoperative GI injury has a mortality rate reported as high as 3.6%.[15] The key to minimizing morbidity with GI injury is understanding risk factors associated with intestinal injury and early recognition. Injury may occur from Veress needle or trocars placement, adhesiolysis, tissue dissection, devascularization injury, and thermal injury. Prior abdominal surgery increases the risk of adhesions to the anterior abdominal wall. In such cases, using an open technique (Hasson method) or gaining access from the left upper quadrant (Palmer point) may be considered; however, even with the proper use of these techniques, intestinal injury may occur.[16,17] Likewise, optical access trocars, designed for additional safety through visualization, also have been associated with GI injury.[18]

Prevention and Detection of GI Injury

It may be difficult to recognize all intestinal injuries intraoperatively during laparotomic or laparoscopic surgery.[16] Injury should be suspected when multiple anterior abdominal wall or intestinal adhesions are present. If there is an unresolved question of intestinal injury, consultation with a surgeon experienced with bowel injury should be obtained. If a small bowel injury is suspected, the bowel should be run with laparoscopic bowel graspers or manually by standard laparotomy until an injury is satisfactorily ruled out. Unrecognized injuries to the intestine usually present with symptoms of nausea, vomiting, anorexia, abdominal pain, and possibly fever by the second to fourth postoperative day.

A meta-analysis of methods used to establish pneumoperitoneum compared open access (Hasson-type) with closed access (needle/trocar) as well as comparing two types of closed access techniques (direct trocar vs needle/trocar).[19] Deaths were only reported in the needle/trocar group rather than the open group. The rarity of death makes it difficult to assess morbidity from these techniques meaningfully. This study was underpowered to adequately compare the two closed techniques. Therefore, the optimal initial port placement has not been definitively determined to date.

Treatment of GI Injury

Intestinal injury may be repaired laparoscopically by surgeons experienced with these types of repairs.[20] It is certainly reasonable to perform a laparotomy to repair an intestinal injury. Performing the appropriate repair should be the focus, rather than aesthetics. In the case of small intestinal injury, the repair should be performed perpendicular to the intestinal axis to lessen the risk of stricture formation. The mucosa and muscularis are typically repaired with a delayed 3-0 absorbable suture. The serosa often is repaired with interrupted 3-0 silk sutures as a second layer. If the laceration to the small bowel exceeds one half of the luminal diameter, segmental resection is recommended.

In the case of thermal injury, a segmental resection is recommended rather than oversewing the defect, as the areas may become necrotic during the healing process resulting in a high incidence of breakdown.

As a general rule, small injuries (2 mm) to the GI tract such as Veress needle injuries, need no repair in the absence of bleeding, and as long as the puncture is not associated with a subsequent rent.[21] In the case of puncture of the large intestine without tearing, nonoperative management with copious irrigation and suction has been suggested.[22]

Large Intestine Issues

The large intestine differs from the small intestine in that its contents have a high bacterial load that puts the patient at higher risk for additional febrile and infectious morbidity. For this reason, it is important to irrigate the peritoneal cavity copiously. Antibiotics also should be given to cover intestinal flora. Trocar injury to the colon is reported to occur with frequency of approximately 1 per 1000 cases.[23] If injury to the rectosigmoid colon is suspected, it may be detected by filling the posterior cul-de-sac with normal saline and performing proctosigmoidoscopy,[24] or by injecting air into the rectum through a catheter-tipped bulb syringe and looking for bubbles (flat tire test).

The management of large intestine injuries depends upon size, site, and length of time to diagnosis. In general, once the diagnosis of colonic injury is made, consultation should be sought with a surgeon who has experience with these types of injuries. In the case of a small rent with minimal soilage, the defect can be closed in two layers with copious irrigation. When a larger injury has occurred and the bowel has not been prepared with a mechanical or antibiotic regimen, or in the case of injuries involving the mesentery, a diverting colostomy is usually necessary. In the case of delayed (postoperative) diagnosis, a diverting colostomy should be performed.

Injury to the Stomach

Relative to small and large bowel injury, there has been little evidence-based literature published about stomach injury during laparoscopy. Based upon survey data, it is estimated that gastric perforation occurs approximately 1 in 3000 cases.[22] As with most surgical injuries, morbidity is directly associated with the size of injury and the length of time between injury and recognition. Risk factors include prior upper abdominal surgery and difficult induction of anesthesia, as a gas distended stomach can lie below the level of the umbilicus. Therefore orogastric or nasogastric suction before Veress needle or trocar placement has been recommended.

Small Veress needle punctures can be treated by irrigation as long as the defect is not bleeding. Larger defects such as trocar injuries require repair by laparoscopy or laparotomy.[25] The defect may be oversewn with a delayed absorbable suture in two layers by a surgeon experienced in gastric surgery. The abdominal cavity should be irrigated and suctioned, being sure to remove any food particles as well as gastric juices. Nasogastric suction usually is maintained postoperatively until normal bowel function returns.

THERMAL BOWEL INJURY

Although safety features have been built into newer laparoscopic equipment, thermal injuries still occur.[26] Thermal injuries are histologically different from traumatic injuries and therefore must be treated differently.[27] Thermal bowel injuries can be differentiated histologically from traumatic injury by the presence of coagulation necrosis and the absence of capillary ingrowth and white cell infiltrate in the former. Because of coagulation necrosis, thermal injuries require wide resection even though the bowel may still have a normal appearance adjacent to the injury, as it may take days for the extent of the injury to become apparent.

REFERENCES

1. Gilmour DT, Dwyer PL, Carey MP. Lower urinary tract injury during gynecologic surgery and its detection by intraoperative cystoscopy. Obstet Gynecol 1999; 94:883–9.
2. Basket TF, Clough H. Perioperative morbidity of hysterectomy for benign gynecological disease. J Obstet Gynaecol 2001;21:504–6.
3. Ibeanu OA, Chesson RR, Echols KT, et al. Urinary tract injury during hysterectomy based on universal cystoscopy. Obstet Gynecol 2009;113:6–10.
4. Gilmour DT, Baskett TF. Disability and litigation from urinary tract injury at benign gynecologic surgery in Canada. Obstet Gynecol 2005;105:109–14.
5. Gill IS, Clayman RV, Albala DM, et al. Retroperitoneal and pelvic extraperitoneal laparoscopy: an international perspective. Urology 1998;52:566–71.
6. Soulie M. Multi-institutional study of complications in 1085 laparoscopic urologic procedures. Urology 2001;58:899–903.
7. Ostrzenski A, Radolinski B, Ostrzenski KM. A review of laparoscopic ureteral injury in pelvic surgery. Obstet Gynecol Surv 2003;58:794–9.
8. Nezhat CH, Seidman DS, Nezhat F, et al. Laparoscopic management of intentional and unintentional cystotomy. J Urol 1996;156:1400–2.
9. Oh BR, Kwon DD, Park KS, et al. Late presentation of ureteral injury after laparoscopic surgery. Obstet Gynecol 2000;95:337–9.
10. Grainger AH, Soderstrom RM, Schiff SF, et al. Ureteral injuries at laparoscopy: insights into diagnosis, management and prevention. Obstet Gynecol 1990;75:839–43.
11. Tulikangas PK, Gill IS, Falcone T. Laparoscopic repair of ureteral injuries. J Am Assoc Gynecol Laparosc 2001;8:259–62.
12. Gilmour DT, Das S, Flowerdew G. Rates of urinary tract injury from gynecologic surgery and the role of intraoperative cystoscopy. Obstet Gynecol 2006;107:1366–72.
13. Smilen SW, Weber AM. ACOG Committee on Practice Bulletins – Gynecology. ACOG Practice Bulletin No. 85: pelvic organ prolapse. Obstet Gynecol 2007; 110:717–29.
14. Brosens I, Gordon A, Campo R, et al. Bowel injury in gynecologic laparoscopy. J Am Assoc Gynecol Laparosc 2003;10:9–13.
15. Van Der Voort M, Heijnsdijk EA, Gouma DJ. Bowel injury as a complication of laparoscopy. Br J Surg 2004;91:1253–8.
16. Vilos GA. Laparoscopic bowel injuries: forty litigated gynaecological cases in Canada. J Obstet Gynaecol Can 2002;24:224–30.
17. Chapron C, Cravello L, Chopin N, et al. Complications during set-up procedures for laparoscopy: open laparoscopy does not reduce the risk of major complications. Acta Obstet Gynecol Scand 2003;82:1125–9.
18. Sharp HT, Dodson MK, Watts DA, et al. Complications associated with optical-access laparoscopic trocars. Obstet Gynecol 2002;99:553–5.
19. Merlin TL, Hiller JE, Maddern GJ, et al. Systematic review of the safety and effectiveness of methods used to establish pneumoperitoneum in laparoscopic surgery. Br J Surg 2003;90:668–79.
20. Nezhat C, Nezhat F, Ambrose W, et al. Laparoscopic repair of small bowel and colon. A report of 26 cases. Surg Endosc 1993;7:88–9.
21. Loffer FD, Pent D. Indications, contraindications and complications of laparoscopy. Obstet Gynecol Surv 1975;30:407–27.

22. Taylor R, Weakley FL, Sullivan BH. Non-operative management of colonic perfo-ration with pneumoperitoneum. Gastrointest Endosc 1978;24:124–5.
23. Krebs HB. Intestinal injury in gynecologic surgery: a ten-year experience. Am J Obstet Gynecol 1986;155:509–14.
24. Nezhat C, Seidman D, Nezhat F, et al. The role of intraoperative proctosig-moidoscopy in laparoscopic pelvic surgery. J Am Assoc Gynecol Laparosc 2004;11:47–9.
25. Spinelli P, Di Felice G, Pizzetti P, et al. Laparoscopic repair of full-thickness stomach injury. Surg Endosc 1991;5:156–7.
26. Chapron C, Pierre F, Harchaoui Y, et al. Gastrointestinal injuries during gynaeco-logical laparoscopy. Hum Reprod 1999;14:333–7.
27. Levy BS, Soderstrom RM, Dail DH. Bowel injuries during laparoscopy. J Reprod Med 1985;30:660–3.

Index

Note: Page numbers of article titles are in **boldface** type

A

Abdomen, lower, major vessels of, at risk during laparoscopy, 388–389
Active electrode injury, 417
Acute compartment syndrome, hysteroscopy and, 401
Alternate path burns, 375–376
Anemia, preoperative management of, in hemorrhage prevention, 429–430
Anesthesia/anesthetics, hysteroscopic complications of, 402–404
Antimicrobial agents, in gynecologic SSI prevention, 380–381
Autologous blood donation, in preoperative management of anemia, 429–430

B

Bipolar currents, 372
Bladder injury, during surgery, 461–462
Bleeding, hysteroscopy and, 414–415
Blended current, 374
Brachial plexus injury, after gynecologic surgery, case example, 452–454
Burn(s)
    alternate path, 375–376
    electrode, in patient, 376
    surgeon, 376–377

C

Capacitance coupling, 376
Carbon dioxide (CO_2), hysteroscopic complications of, 406
Cephalosporin(s), in gynecological SSI prevention, 380–381
Closed laparoscopy, instrument insertion during, vessel injury prevention during, 389–392
CO_2. See *Carbon dioxide (CO_2)*.
CO_2 insufflators, hysteroscopic complications of, 408
Coagulation currents, 372–373
Common peroneal nerve injury, after gynecologic surgery, case example, 457
Current(s). See specific types.
Current diversion, 417–418
Cut currents, 372–373

D

Desiccation, 374–375
Distending agents, hysteroscopic complications of, 406–410
    background of, 406
    CO_2, 406
    CO_2 insufflators–related, 408

Obstet Gynecol Clin N Am 37 (2010) 469–474
doi:10.1016/S0889-8545(10)00077-X
0889-8545/10/$ – see front matter © 2010 Elsevier Inc. All rights reserved.

Moving?

Make sure your subscription moves with you!

To notify us of your new address, find your **Clinics Account Number** (located on your mailing label above your name), and contact customer service at:

Email: journalscustomerservice-usa@elsevier.com

800-654-2452 (subscribers in the U.S. & Canada)
314-447-8871 (subscribers outside of the U.S. & Canada)

Fax number: 314-447-8029

Elsevier Health Sciences Division
Subscription Customer Service
3251 Riverport Lane
Maryland Heights, MO 63043

*To ensure uninterrupted delivery of your subscription, please notify us at least 4 weeks in advance of move.

Printed and bound by CPI Group (UK) Ltd, Croydon, CR0 4YY

03/10/2024

01040459-0013